Daniela Much

Nutritional fatty acids during pregnancy & lactation

Daniela Much

Nutritional fatty acids during pregnancy & lactation

Do they play a role as a prevention strategy against childhood overweight in early life?

Südwestdeutscher Verlag für Hochschulschriften

Impressum / Imprint
Bibliografische Information der Deutschen Nationalbibliothek: Die Deutsche Nationalbibliothek verzeichnet diese Publikation in der Deutschen Nationalbibliografie; detaillierte bibliografische Daten sind im Internet über http://dnb.d-nb.de abrufbar.
Alle in diesem Buch genannten Marken und Produktnamen unterliegen warenzeichen-, marken- oder patentrechtlichem Schutz bzw. sind Warenzeichen oder eingetragene Warenzeichen der jeweiligen Inhaber. Die Wiedergabe von Marken, Produktnamen, Gebrauchsnamen, Handelsnamen, Warenbezeichnungen u.s.w. in diesem Werk berechtigt auch ohne besondere Kennzeichnung nicht zu der Annahme, dass solche Namen im Sinne der Warenzeichen- und Markenschutzgesetzgebung als frei zu betrachten wären und daher von jedermann benutzt werden dürften.

Bibliographic information published by the Deutsche Nationalbibliothek: The Deutsche Nationalbibliothek lists this publication in the Deutsche Nationalbibliografie; detailed bibliographic data are available in the Internet at http://dnb.d-nb.de.
Any brand names and product names mentioned in this book are subject to trademark, brand or patent protection and are trademarks or registered trademarks of their respective holders. The use of brand names, product names, common names, trade names, product descriptions etc. even without a particular marking in this works is in no way to be construed to mean that such names may be regarded as unrestricted in respect of trademark and brand protection legislation and could thus be used by anyone.

Coverbild / Cover image: www.ingimage.com

Verlag / Publisher:
Südwestdeutscher Verlag für Hochschulschriften
ist ein Imprint der / is a trademark of
OmniScriptum GmbH & Co. KG
Heinrich-Böcking-Str. 6-8, 66121 Saarbrücken, Deutschland / Germany
Email: info@svh-verlag.de

Herstellung: siehe letzte Seite /
Printed at: see last page
ISBN: 978-3-8381-3796-4

Zugl. / Approved by: München, Technische Universität München, Dissertation, 2013

Copyright © 2014 OmniScriptum GmbH & Co. KG
Alle Rechte vorbehalten. / All rights reserved. Saarbrücken 2014

This study is based on the following papers, referred to in the text by Roman numerals I-IV

I. Hauner H, **Much D**, Vollhardt C, Brunner S, Schmid D, Sedlmeier EM, Heimberg E, Schuster T, Zimmermann A, Schneider KT, Bader BL, Amann-Gassner U. Effect of reducing the n-6:n-3 long-chain polyunsaturated fatty acid (LCPUFA) ratio during pregnancy and lactation on infant adipose tissue growth within the first year of life (INFAT-study): an open-label, randomized, controlled trial.
Am J Clin Nutr. 2012 Feb; 95(2):383-94. Epub 2011 Dec 28.

II. **Much D**, Brunner S, Vollhardt C, Schmid D, Sedlmeier EM, Brüderl M, Heimberg E, Bartke N, Boehm G, Bader BL, Amann-Gassner U, Hauner H. Effect of dietary intervention to reduce the n-6/n-3 fatty acid ratio on maternal and fetal fatty acid profile and its relation to offspring growth and body composition at 1 year of age.
Eur J Clin Nutr. 2013 Mar; 67(3):282-8. Epub 2013 Jan 23; poster presentation at ISSFAL 2012.

III. **Much D**, Brunner S, Vollhardt C, Schmid D, Sedlmeier EM, Brüderl M, Heimberg E, Bartke N, Boehm G, Bader BL, Amann-Gassner U, Hauner H. Breast-milk fatty acid profile in relation to infant growth and body composition - results from the INFAT-study.
Pediatr Res. 2013 May; Epub ahead of print: doi: 10.1038/pr.2013.82.; oral presentation at ISSFAL 2012.

IV. **Much D**, Heimberg E, Brunner S, Vollhardt C, Schmid D, Brüderl M, Amann-Gassner U, Hauner H. Sonographic assessment of abdominal fat distribution within the first year of life in relation to skinfold thickness measurements and anthropometry- results from the INFAT-study.

(*manuscript drafted*)

TABLE OF CONTENTS

1	INTRODUCTION	1
1.1	Childhood obesity- a growing epidemic?	3
1.2	New ways towards obesity prevention	4
1.3	Early infancy- a critical period for the onset of obesity	5
1.4	Early adipose tissue growth in men	6
1.5	The role of LCPUFAs in adipose tissue development	9
1.5.1	N-6/n-3 fatty acid ratio and childhood obesity: epidemiological data	9
1.5.2	N-6/n-3 fatty acid ratio and adipose tissue development: in vitro and animal studies	10
1.5.3	Fish oil/LCPUFAs supplementation and adipose tissue development in the offspring- Human trials	12
2	AIMS OF THE THESIS	16
3	SUBJECTS AND METHODS	19
3.1	Study design	19
3.2	Recruitment	19
3.3	Inclusion and exclusion criteria	19
3.4	Screening examination	I5
3.5	Randomization, data management, and ethical requirements	21
3.6	Study groups and intervention	22
3.7	Adverse events	23
3.8	Dietary intake	23
3.9	Blood and breast milk sampling	23
3.10	Fatty acid analysis in plasma phospholipids (PLs), red blood cells (RBCs) and breast milk	24
3.11	Compliance	26

3.12	Infant growth and development	27
3.13	Infant fat mass and fat distribution assessed by SFT	27
3.14	Infant fat mass and fat distribution assessed by ultrasonography	28
3.15	Evaluation of the ultrasound images	32
3.16	Blinding of participants and study team	36
3.17	Statistical analysis	36
4	**RESULTS**	**38**
4.1	Clinical data and comparison of the randomized groups	38
4.1.1	Participant characteristics	38
4.1.2	Compliance	38
4.1.3	Blood coagulation and tolerance	43
4.1.4	Pregnancy outcomes and complications	43
4.1.5	Infant growth	45
4.1.6	Infant fat mass and distribution	48
4.1.7	Subgroup analysis	54
4.2	Maternal and cord blood fatty acid profile in relation to infant body composition	55
4.2.1	Sample collection	55
4.2.2	Maternal fatty acid profile over the course of pregnancy and lactation	55
4.2.3	Cord blood fatty acid profile	56
4.2.4	Relationship between maternal fatty acid profile at 32nd week of gestation and cord blood fatty acid profile	61
4.2.5	Relationship between maternal LCPUFAs profile and pregnancy duration	62
4.2.6	Maternal LCPUFAs profile in relation to infant growth parameters and fat mass	62

4.2.7	Neonatal LCPUFAs in relation to infant growth parameters and fat mass	67
4.3	Breast milk fatty acid profile in relation to infant body composition	69
4.3.1	Sample Collection	69
4.3.2	Maternal breast milk fatty acid profile over the course of lactation	69
4.3.3	Relationship between the fatty acid composition of breast milk and maternal blood	72
4.3.4	Infant blood fatty acid profile in RBCs	73
4.3.5	Relationship between the fatty acid composition of breast milk and infant RBCs	75
4.3.6	Relationship between breast milk fatty acid profile and infant growth and body composition	75
4.4	Sonographic assessment of infant body composition in relation to anthropometry and skinfold thickness measurement	81
4.4.1	Precision of ultrasonography	81
4.4.2	Adipose tissue growth by age and group	84
4.4.3	Differences in adipose tissue growth in boys and girls	85
4.4.4	Correlation coefficients of the different measures of fat mass	89
5	**DISCUSSION**	**95**
5.1	Clinical results (Paper I)	95
5.2	Maternal and cord blood fatty acid profile in relation to infant body composition (Paper II)	100
5.3	Breast milk fatty acid profile in relation to infant body composition (Paper III)	107
5.4	Sonographic assment of fat mass and fat distribution and its relation to anthropometry and skinfold thickness measurements (Paper IV)	115

5.4.1	Method and reproducibility	115
5.4.2	Adipose tissue development and sex differences	121
5.4.3	Correlations of the different fat measures	123
6	**CONCLUSION AND FURTHER PERSPECTIVES**	**126**
7	**SUMMARY**	**132**
8	**ACKNOWLEDGEMENTS**	**135**

APPENDIX	**137**
REFERENCES	**144**

TABLE OF FIGURES

Figure 1: Overview about n-3 LCPUFAs supplementation trials 15
Figure 2: Sensitive phases of adipose tissue development and possible impact of LCPUFAs. 18
Figure 3: Study design 20
Figure 4: SFT measurement at 6 weeks pp 27
Figure 5: Holtain Caliper 27
Figure 6: Sonographic investigation at 6 weeks pp 29
Figure 7: 10-MHz linear probe 29
Figure 8: Sonographic assessment in sagittal direction 30
Figure 9: Examples for demonstration of the holding technique in sagittal plane. 30
Figure 10: Sonographic assessment in axial direction 31
Figure 11: Examples for the holding technique in the axial plane 31
Figure 12: Example for measurements in the sagittal plane 32
Figure 13: Example of a measurement in the axial plane 33
Figure 14: Thin subcutaneous fat layer 34
Figure 15: Medium thickness of subcutaneous fat layer 35
Figure 16: Large thickness of subcutaneous fat layer 35
Figure 17: Flow Chart of the INFAT-study 41
Figure 18: Growth pattern of the infants from birth up to 1 year of life. ... 47
Figure 19: Individual SFT during the first year of life. 51
Figure 20: Infant body composition assessed by SFT during the first year of life. 52
Figure 21: Development of abdominal subcutaneous and preperitoneal fat mass over the first year of life 54
Figure 22: Relationship of the different fat measures among each other stratified by time point of the investigation 94

Figure 23: Examples of measuring subcutaneous and preperitoneal fat layers in different breathing phases 118
Figure 24: Examples (down with marked labeling) for demonstration of the different within-echo (arrow) within the subcutaneous adipose tissue (yellow areal) and for different echogenecity of preperitoneal fat tissue (red areal) with increasingly higher echogenicity in the left picture. 119

LIST OF TABLES

Table 1: Characteristics of the study population at baseline 40

Table 2: Women's compliance with the fish oil intake and the AA-balanced diet 42

Table 3: Birth outcomes and complications 44

Table 4: Growth pattern and growth indices from birth up to 1 year of life 46

Table 5: Adipose tissue growth and subcutaneous fat distribution during the first year of life assessed by skinfold thickness measurements 50

Table 6: Adipose tissue growth and abdominal fat distribution during the first year of life assessed by ultrasonography[1] 53

Table 7: Maternal RBCs fatty acid profile 58

Table 8: Cord blood plasma PLs and RBCs fatty acid profile 59

Table 9: Cord blood RBCs fatty acid profile according to gender 60

Table 10: Correlation coefficients between A) maternal RBCs fatty acid profile at 32nd week of gestation and cord blood RBCs fatty acid profile and B) maternal plasma PLs fatty acid profile at 32nd week of gestation and cord blood plasma PLs 61

Table 11: Final adjusted multiple regression analysis and partial correlation coefficients on the effect of maternal RBCs fatty acid profile (at 32nd week of gestation) on infant growth and growth indices 64

Table 12: Final adjusted multiple regression analysis and partial correlation coefficients on the effect of maternal RBCs fatty acid profile (at 32nd week of gestation) on infant adipose tissue growth assessed by skinfold thickness measurements 65

Table 13: Final adjusted multiple regression analysis and partial correlation coefficients on the effect of maternal RBCs fatty acid status (at 32nd week of gestation) on infant adipose tissue growth assessed by ultrasonography 66

Table 14: Final adjusted multiple regression model and partial correlation coefficients on the effect of cord blood RBCs fatty acid status on infant growth and body fat mass at birth 68

Table 15: Breast milk fatty acid profile 71

Table 16: Correlation coefficients between breast milk LCPUFAs and the respective LCPUFAs in maternal plasma PLs and RBCs 72

Table 17: Infant RBCs fatty acid profile 74

Table 18: Correlation coefficients between breast milk LCPUFAs and the respective LCPUFAs in infant plasma PLs and RBCs 75

Table 19: Final adjusted multiple regression analysis and partial correlation coefficients on the effect of maternal breast milk n-3 fatty acid profile at early (6th week pp) lactation on infant body composition 79

Table 20: Final adjusted multiple regression analysis and partial correlation coefficients on the effect of maternal breast milk n-6 fatty acid profile at early lactation (6th week pp) on infant growth and growth indices over the 1st year of life 80

Table 21: Error of precision, shown as EP_{RMS} in % of fat thicknesses measured and as areas for all infants in their age group, respectively. 82

Table 22: Intraclass-correlation-coefficients (ICC) of the precision measurements for all infants in each age group 83

Table 23: Percentage interobserver-difference shown as EP_{RMS} in % of average fat thicknesses and areas (n=45 infants) 84

Table 24: Sex differences in anthropometry and adipose tissue growth assessed 87

Table 25: Sex differences in adipose tissue growth and fat distribution assessed by ultrasonography 88

Table 26: Spearman-correlation-coefficients for anthropometric measures 90

Table 27: Spearman-correlation coefficients of the sonographic measures 91

Table 28: Spearman-correlation coefficients of the different fat measures 93

ABBREVATIONS

AA	Arachidonic acid (C20:4n-6)
Aax sc	Sonographic assessment of adipose tissue, axial plane, Area of subcutaneous fat
ALA	α-linolenic acid (C18:3n-3)
APGAR-score	Score to assess the condition of a newborn after birth (1-10)
Asag pp	Sonographic assessment of adipose tissue, sagittal plane, Area preperitoneal fat
Asag sc	Sonographic assessment of adipose tissue, sagittal plane, Area subcutaneous fat
ax l	Sonographic assessment of adipose tissue, axial plane, thickness of subcutaneous fat layer, 1 cm left of linea alba
ax m	Sonographic assessment of adipose tissue, axial plane, thickness of subcutaneous fat layer, on the top of linea alba
ax r	Sonographic assessment of adipose tissue, axial plane, thickness of subcutaneous fat layer, 1cm right of linea alba
BMI	Body Mass Index
CT	Computer tomography
DEXA	Dual-Energy-X-Ray-Absorptiometry
DGE	Deutsche Gesellschaft für Ernährung (German Nutrition Society)
DHA	Docosahexaenoic acid (C22:6n-3)
DHγLA	Dihomo gamma linolenic acid (C20:3n-6)
DPA	Docosapentaenoic acid (C22:5n-3)
DOHaD	Developmental Origins of Health and Disease

EDTA	Ethylene diamine tetraacetic acid
EPA	Eicosapentaenoic acid (C20:5n-3)
FA	Fatty acid
FAME	Fatty acid methyl esters
GDM	Gestational diabetes mellitus
GLC	Gas liquid chromatography
HAPO-study	Hyperglycemia and adverse pregnancy outcome study
ICC	Intraclass-correlation-coefficient, precision of the measurement
INFAT	Impact of Nutritional Fatty acids during pregnancy and lactation for early human Adipose Tissue development
KiGGS	Kinder- und Jugendgesundheitssurvey
LA	Linoleic acid (C18:2n-6)
LCPUFAs	Long chain polyunsaturated fatty acids
M.	Musculus
MHz	Megahertz
mo	month
MRI	Magnetic resonance imaging
MUFA	Monounsaturated fatty acid
n-3 LCPUFAs	Omega-3 long chain poly unsaturated fatty acids
n-6 LCPUFAs	Omega-6 long chain polyunsaturated fatty acids
n.s.	not significant
PF_{RMS}	Error of precision, calculated as „root mean square" of individual coefficients of variation
PG	Prostaglandin
PGI_2	Prostacyclin
pp	postpartum

PP	Preperitoneal
PPAR	Peroxisome proliferator-activated receptor
PUFA	Polyunsaturated fatty acids
RBCs	Red blood cells
RCT	Randomized Controlled Trial
R PP/SC	Sonographic assessment of adipose tissue, Ratio preperitoneal fat/subcutaneous fat
sc	subcutaneous
sag caudal pp	Sonographic assessment of adipose tissue, sagittal plane, caudal thickness of preperitoneal fat layer
sag caudal sc	Sonographic assessment of adipose tissue, sagittal plane, caudal thickness of subcutaneous fat layer
sag cranial pp	Sonographic assessment of adipose tissue, sagittal plane cranial thickness of preperitoneal fat layer
sag cranial sc	Sonographic assessment of adipose tissue, sagittal plane, cranial thickness of subcutaneous fat layer
SD	Standarddeviation
SAFA	Saturated fatty acid
SFT	Skinfold thickness measurement
US	United States
wk gest	Week of gestation
WHO	World Health Organisation
WC	Waist circumference
y	year

1 INTRODUCTION

The global rise in childhood obesity over the past decades has reached an epidemic scale. Effective primary prevention strategies are essential to combat the disease that, once manifested, has been shown to be particularly resistant to therapy (World Health Organization 2009).

A growing body of evidence, which is predominantly based on experimental studies in mammals (Taylor and Poston 2007), has provided useful leads toward pregnancy and lactation as a new period for primary prevention of obesity because it was shown that the nutritional environment a fetus experiences in utero may have a critical impact on the health of the developing offspring in the long term (Gluckman and Hanson 2008).

High maternal energy or fat intake per se (Armitage et al. 2005) and the ingestion of specific fatty acids during the gestation and suckling period appears to be critical for adipose tissue development of rodents (Azain 2004) with a reduced dietary ratio of n-6 to n-3 LCPUFAs decreasing fat cell differentiation and fat deposition (Massiera et al. 2003; Ailhaud and Guesnet 2004).

However, the composition of fatty acids in the diet in industrialized countries and, hence, the diet of pregnant women, has substantially shifted toward an increasing dominance of n-6 compared with n-3 LCPUFAs over the past decades, which is also reflected in the composition of fatty acids in breast milk (Ailhaud et al. 2006).

This observation brought up the hypothesis that a reduced dietary n-6/n-3 fatty acid ratio during early critical windows of fat cell development may limit adipose tissue growth and, thereby, may offer a novel strategy for the primary prevention of childhood obesity (Ailhaud and Guesnet 2004).

Although supplementation with n-3 LCPUFAs during pregnancy and lactation has become popular because of reported beneficial effects on the neurodevelopment of the infant (Helland et al. 2003; Dunstan et al. 2008; Jensen et al. 2005), data on the potential role of n-3 LCPUFAs in influencing fat mass in humans are scarce. As recently reviewed by Muhlhausler et al (Muhlhausler et al. 2010), few post hoc analyses of studies that addressed this issue have shown variable and inconclusive results. None of the trials was designed to assess infant fat mass as the primary outcome.

Aim of the present study, the INFAT-study (*I*mpact of *N*utritional *F*atty acids during pregnancy and lactation for early human *A*dipose *T*issue development) was to examine the effect of a reduction in the n-6/n-3 LCPUFAs ratio in the diet of pregnant women and breastfeeding mothers on adipose tissue growth in their infants´ ≤1 y of age by using 2 methods of body fat assessment, skinfold thickness measurement and abdominal ultrasonography. Besides the comparison of the randomized groups, we additionally aimed to explore the potential association between maternal, cord blood and breast milk LCPUFAs and infant adipose tissue growth in the whole study population. Moreover ultrasonography as a new body composition technique in infants´ ≤ 1 year of age was tested and cross-validated with anthropometry and SFT measurements. A detailed description of the study design and rationale has been published (Hauner et al. 2009; Hauner et al. 2012).

1.1 Childhood obesity- a growing epidemic?

Historically, a heavy child meant a healthy child, and the concept "the bigger the better" was widely accepted. Today, this perception has dramatically changed on the basis of evidence that childhood obesity is associated with a wide range of serious health complications affecting vascular and metabolic functions and the fact that the disease has reached epidemic dimensions on a global level (Ebbeling et al. 2002; de Onis et al. 2010).

The most recent estimates of obesity prevalence rates in United States (US) children and adolescents for 2009-2010 from the National Health and Nutrition Examination Survey reported 16.9% of US children and adolescents being obese (Ogden et al. 2012). Current prevalence estimates for Germany based on the KiGGS survey (Kinder- und Jugendgesundheitssurvey) (Kurth and Schaffrath 2010), found 14.8% of the children and adolescents in Germany aged 2-17 years being overweight, including 6.1% suffering from obesity (according to the Kromeyer-Hauschild reference system)(Kromeyer-Hauschild et al. 2001). In absolute numbers referring to the most recent population numbers, this corresponds to 1.7 million overweight children and adolescents in Germany aged 2 years and older, 750.000 of whom are obese (Kurth and Schaffrath 2010).

A meta-analysis of 154 historical studies by Olds moreover described very unfavorable changes in the body composition of young people from developed countries: over the period from 1951 to 2003, the triceps and subscapular skinfold thicknesses have increased by 0.4–0.5 mm per decade, percentage body fat increased by 0.9% per decade and the fat distribution in the 0-18 year olds has become a more centralized patterning (Olds 2009).

In 2008 Wang et al. estimated that the prevalence of obesity among US children will reach 30% by 2030 (Wang et al. 2008), however, very recent statistics rather suggest that the prevalence rate of childhood obesity might be leveling off in developed countries. Stable prevalence rates have been reported for US children and adolescents (Ogden et al. 2012) and even declining proportions were observed in German children starting school (Moss et al. 2012).

It was suggested that the measures made towards prevention and treatment of obesity in the past, most of them initiated in the 1990s and implemented afterwards (World Health Organization 2009), could have contributed to this positive development (Ogden et al. 2012; Moss et al. 2012).

1.2 New ways towards obesity prevention

The number of preventive actions that governments, communities and families can implement to control obesity and promote health has been aggregating, but the international evidence base remains unclear to date. Current attempts to control the threat by community- or familybased prevention strategies provided limited data on the quality and effectiveness of such programs and thus do not allow for generalizability (Campbell et al. 2001). In view of the tremendous obesity epidemic there is an urgent need to develop and evaluate new approaches to address this issue.

In recent years, evidence was accumulating that some environmental factors in utero (i.e. dietary factors during pregnancy) may have a programming effect on lifelong health of the child and thereby also could influence the propensity to develop obesity (Oken and Gillman 2003; Gillman et al. 2008). This observation brought up the DOHaD concept (<u>D</u>evelopmental <u>O</u>rigins of <u>H</u>ealth <u>a</u>nd <u>D</u>isease) proposing that many diseases originate through an unbalanced nutrition *in utero* and during early infancy. It was supposed that the perinatal period, a phase of rapid growth, might offer an important period for the application of prevention strategies against childhood obesity as it represents a life phase in which the individual's susceptibility for later obesity development is determined (Gluckman and Hanson 2008).

1.3 Early infancy- a critical period for the onset of obesity

The rapidly increasing rates of childhood and adulthood obesity urgently need a better insight into the levels of persistence of high body mass index (BMI) over the life span.

Various data have demonstrated that early infancy constitutes a critical period for the onset of obesity (Peneau et al. 2011; Baird et al. 2005; Gillman 2010). Obese children may be at risk for long-term tracking of obesity to adulthood (Pietilainen et al. 2001; Singh et al. 2008; Wright et al. 2010).

Baird et al. carried out a systematic review of 24 studies to assess the association between infant growth and subsequent obesity (Baird et al. 2005). They considered infants with a certain pattern of growth at increased risk of subsequent obesity, e.g. infants who are at the highest end of the distribution for weight or BMI or infants who grow very rapidly during infancy.

These data were also confirmed by results of the Project Viva, an ongoing prospective US cohort study, which showed that more-rapid increases in weight-for-length in the first 6 months of life were associated with sharply increased risk of obesity at 3 years of age (Taveras et al. 2009).

Similarly, a French study in 1582 children showed the simultaneous association of large infant weight and BMI attained at 1 year of age, and early rapid infant growth (average monthly weight gain) along with overweight at 7–9 years, as well as involvement of early growth velocity variations, retrospectively (Peneau et al. 2011).

These data collectively showed that it is especially the changes in weight status in infancy ("early weight gain") which may influence the risk of becoming obese later on, more than weight status at birth alone (Peneau et al. 2011).

Recent findings of the so-called "Generation R study", a prospective cohort study from the Netherlands, provided further data on this topic. They found that rapid growth rates during both, *fetal life* and infancy are associated with increased abdominal subcutaneous and preperitoneal fat mass, the latter considered to be a proxy for intra-abdominal fat mass, in 481 healthy children at 2 years of age (Durmus et al. 2010). To understand pregnancy and the early postpartum period, thus early infancy, as a key period for human adipogenesis it is necessary to provide information on fat cell development in humans.

1.4 Early adipose tissue growth in men

To date, the development of white adipose tissue in human fetal life has been poorly studied. However, from histological studies it is known, that the first traces of adipose tissue are detectable in the human fetus between the 14th and 16th week of gestation (n=488) (Poissonnet et al. 1984). Fat lobules are the earliest structures to be identified before typical fat cells appear. After the 23rd week of gestation the total number of fat lobules remains approximately constant and from the 23rd to 29th week the growth of adipose tissue is determined mainly by an increase in size of the lobules (Poissonnet et al. 1983). Adipose tissue becomes noticeable at first in the head and the neck, later in the trunk, and finally in the upper and lower limbs of the fetus (Poissonnet et al. 1984).

Humans differ from most mammals by depositing significant quantities of body fat mass already in utero. More than 90 % of the fetal fat deposition occurs in the last 10 weeks of pregnancy (Haggarty 2002). Western infants accrete fatty acids in the order of LA>AA>DHA at all stages during pregnancy. The highest accretion rates are reached in the last 5 weeks of gestation, i.e. 342 mg LA, 95 mg AA and 42 mg DHA/day. At term, most of the infant's LA, AA and DHA is located in adipose tissue (68, 44 and 50%, respectively)(Kuipers et al. 2012).

The human baby is born with a body fat content of 13-15 % of total body mass, mainly distributed in subcutaneous regions (Hauner et al. 2012; Widdowsen 1950). Immediately after birth, body fat mass increases from 13% up to 20 % at the age of 1 year assessed by skinfold thickness measurement (Hauner et al. 2012). About 40 – 65 % of body weight gain during the first 6 months is accounted for by body fat deposition (Fomon et al. 1982; McLaren 1987). This increase in fat mass is mainly due to an enlargement of existing fat cell size (Ailhaud G 2004; Hager et al. 1977; Sjostrom and William-Olsson 1981).

There are some older studies suggesting that early life stages can be seen as critical periods for fat cell development and adipose tissue growth in humans (reviewed in Hauner et al., in press):

A high proliferation and differentiation capacity of cells isolated from early fat depots has been reported which may contribute to define the space for later adipose tissue expansion. This acquisition of fat cells early in life appears to be an irreversible process (Ailhaud G 2004). The early determination of fat cell number was confirmed by an elegant study using an isotope technique (Spalding et al. 2008). This study further described an annual turnover rate of fat cells of about 10% at all ages and levels of body mass index by analyzing the integrated 14C from nuclear bomb tests performed between 1955 and 1963 in genomic DNA.

Adipose tissue growth and cellularity varies between different age groups and sex. Sensitive developmental periods occur directly after birth and between 9 and 13 years (Salans et al. 1973). This hypothesis was confirmed some years later (Baum et al. 1986), measuring the highest thymidine kinase activity as an index of cellular proliferation in infants during the first year of life and as a second peak in the preadolescent stage. In a large cohort study, 2-year old children showed a small but continuous increase in both fat cell size and number during early childhood over a period of four years (Knittle et al. 1979). Interestingly, also later in vitro studies have shown that stromal adipocyte precursor cells from human adipose tissue exhibit the highest proliferation and differentiation capacity during the first year of life and at prepuberty also supporting the concept of sensitive periods of adipose tissue growth early in life (Hauner and Wabitsch 1989).

1.5 The role of LCPUFAs in adipose tissue development

Recently the role of LCPUFAs in adipose tissue development was re-evaluated in the latest review by our working group. A draft of the manuscript, containing the main epidemiological data, *in vitro* and animal studies as well as human trials which link obesity in the offspring with altered n-6/n-3 fatty acid ratio, has been accepted for publication in the AJCN (Hauner et. al., in press).

1.5.1 N-6/n-3 fatty acid ratio and childhood obesity: epidemiological data

More indirect evidence for a role of the fatty acid composition in human adipose tissue development can be deduced from epidemiological data, showing that the n-6/n-3 fatty acid ratio in the diet of industrialized countries has changed considerable towards an increasing dominance of n-6 fatty acids over recent decades (Sanders 2000; Kris-Etherton et al. 2000; Blasbalg et al. 2011).

These dietary changes are also reflected in the fatty acid pattern of breast milk, in particular regarding the linoleic/ alpha-linolenic acid (LA/ALA) ratio. Between 1945 and 1995 the content of LA in breast milk from US women has steadily increased from ~7 to ~16% of total fatty acids, whereas the percentage of ALA has remained essentially unchanged with approximately 1% of total fatty acids. Consequently, the ratio of LA/ALA has progressively increased to reach a mean value of 16:1 breast milk in US women, which is 50% higher than those of European women (Sanders 2000).These observations coupled with increasing rates of childhood overweight and obesity over the same time period give further support to a potential link between the dietary fatty acid composition and the development of infant adipose tissue development (Ailhaud et al. 2006; Ailhaud and Guesnet 2004).

1.5.2 N-6/n-3 fatty acid ratio and adipose tissue development: in vitro and animal studies

In vitro studies have provided convincing evidence that the balance of n-6 versus n-3 fatty acids plays an important role in critical phases of adipose tissue development. In particular, it was shown that the n-6 fatty acid arachidonic acid inhibits cell proliferation and promotes differentiation to adipocytes in the preadipocyte stage mediated through action of its metabolite prostacyclin (Ailhaud et al. 2006; Massiera et al. 2003), whereas the n-3 LCPUFAs DHA and EPA rather counteract this process (Ailhaud et al. 2006; Massiera et al. 2003; Azain 2004; Madsen et al. 2005). Furthermore, the n-3 fatty acids were also shown to act on mature adipocytes in the process of lipid storage and accumulation (Madsen et al. 2005).

The underlying mechanisms include effects on the regulation of transcription factors representing key molecules for both adipocyte differentiation (e.g. PPAR gamma and C/EBPs) and lipogenesis (e.g. SREP-1c), which are mediated either by the fatty acid per se or their active metabolites such as prostaglandins (Azain 2004; Madsen et al. 2005).

Furthermore, there is good agreement from animal studies for anti-obesity effects of n-3 LCPUFAs supplementation as evidenced by decreased cellularity of adipose tissue (Flachs et al. 2009) and reduced lipid synthesis (Arai et al. 2009) suggesting a role for n-3 fatty acid in reducing both hyperplasia as well as hypertrophy in growing fat depots.

More recently, attention was shifted towards the potential programming effect of modifying the fatty acid composition in the maternal diet during the gestation/suckling period on offspring obesity.

However, a recent systematic review of animal studies, investigating the effects of increased n-3 LCPUFAs supply during pregnancy and lactation on offspring body composition, concluded that there is insufficient evidence to date to definitely evaluate the role of pre- and early postnatal maternal n-3 LCPUFAs supplementation on offspring fat mass development (Muhlhausler et al. 2011b). In particular, there is considerable disparity among the available studies in terms of the type of intervention (n-3 LCPUFAs or ALA), the time window the intervention was applied, the mode and time-point of adiposity assessment, the nature of the control group and study quality.

The fact that most studies did not restrict the intervention to the prenatal and early postnatal period, but continued the exposure after weaning, makes it difficult to disentangle potential effects of increased n-3 LCPUFAs supply on developing fat depots in utero (such as reduced proliferation and differentiation of adipocytes) compared to effects occurring after birth (e.g. suppression of fat storage). A more recent study in which the n-3 LCPUFAs exposure was limited to the perinatal period and the pubs were weaned to a standard diet, observed an increased percentage of body fat, particularly through accumulation of subcutaneous fat depots, in the offspring of mothers fed the n-3 LCPUFAs enriched diet, without affecting the expression of major genes regulating key steps in adipogenesis and lipogenesis (Muhlhausler et al. 2011a). In contrast, another study established a model of postnatal programming through increased n-3 LCPUFAs supply and reported reduced fat accumulation in the offspring in adult life after a western style diet, together with healthier plasma lipid and glucose homeostasis and less hypertrophic adipocytes. These results emphasize that early postnatal nutrition has a programming effect on body composition and metabolism (Oosting et al. 2010).

These conflicting results suggest that nutritional influences during different phases of perinatal development (prenatal vs. early postnatal period) might confer different susceptibility towards increased fat storage and highlight the need for further studies addressing this issue. Moreover, effects might also differ depending on the macronutrient composition and overall quality of the diet and it appears conceivable that n-3 LCPUFAs might exert preventive actions especially under exposure to a high-fat western diet.

1.5.3 Fish oil/LCPUFAs supplementation and adipose tissue development in the offspring- Human trials

The biological plausibility based on these observations together with the increasing awareness for the perinatal period as a sensitive period when nutritional influences could have long-lasting impact on future health, led to the hypothesis that altering the fatty acid composition in maternal nutrition during pregnancy and lactation could have a significant programming effect on body composition in the offspring (Massiera et al. 2003).

The first randomized controlled trials (RCT) involving supplementation with n-3 LCPUFAs during pregnancy were focusing largely on pregnancy outcome and infant neurodevelopment, whereas the effect of increased n-3 LCPUFAs exposure on infant body composition has only recently received attention. To date, this upcoming research question has almost exclusively been addressed in post-hoc analyses of studies which were originally designed to assess other infant outcomes. As recently reviewed by Muhlhausler et al., four retrospective analyses of three RCTs addressed the potential role of perinatal n-3 LCPUFAs supplementation on body composition in infancy and childhood and came to rather inconclusive results (Muhlhausler et al. 2010). Since publication of this systematic review, two analyses of another RCT, the NUHEAL trial, comparing the effects of maternal fish oil supplementation, folate or both, reported results on BMI as a secondary outcome, but again observed no differences in children´s BMI at 4 and at 6.5 years, respectively, between the groups (Escolano-Margarit et al. 2011; Campoy et al. 2011) (**Figure 1**). Recently, a six-year follow-up study of German children whose mothers received a supplement of 200mg/day DHA from midpregnancy through 3 months of lactation no longer found a lower BMI in the supplemented group compared with the control group (Bergmann et al. 2012) as previously observed at 21 months of age (Bergmann et al. 2007).

When aggregating the findings, the high variability of these studies regarding the timing and duration of the intervention (pregnancy and/or lactation), the dosage of n-3 LCPUFAs supplementation, compliance and other methodological aspects has to be considered (Muhlhausler et al. 2010). Of note, most studies relied on rather indirect growth parameters such as BMI or BMI z-scores and in only one study skinfold thickness measurements were performed to determine percentage body fat and, thus, to discriminate between fat and lean body mass (Lauritzen et al. 2005a; Asserhoj et al. 2009). Consequently, these inconsistent results do not allow a definite and firm conclusion on the role of n-3 LCPUFAs during the perinatal period by supplementing pregnant women/lactating mothers in determining offspring adiposity development.

The only study to date with a follow-up period up to adolescence/early adulthood was recently published and found no difference in BMI, waist circumference and selected biochemical parameters between offspring of mothers supplemented with fish oil compared to the control group at the age of 19 years, clearly arguing against a long-term effect of fish oil supplementation during pregnancy on offspring adiposity in adolescence (Rytter et al. 2012).

The first RCT to investigate the effect of n-3 LCPUFAs vs. n-6 LCPUFAs intake during the first 9-18 months of *infancy* on adipose tissue growth, found no association between fish oil consumption relative to sunflower oil consumption and any of the anthropometric measures related to the size of the fat mass (z-Scores SFT) in the completing 133 infants, but a lower triceps-to-subscapular skinfold ratio at 18 mo was reported in the infants from the fish oil group (Andersen et al. 2012).

This limited data highlights the need for prospective RCTs investigating the impact of a perinatal reduction of the n-6/n-3 LCPUFAs ratio on infant adipose tissue growth, involving longitudinal assessments of infant body composition. Hereby, the greatest challenge is the use of sensitive and well established techniques for measuring body composition as precisely as possible over the life-course, particularly during childhood and adolescence.

Figure 1: Overview about n-3 LCPUFAs supplementation trials (Hauner et al., in press)

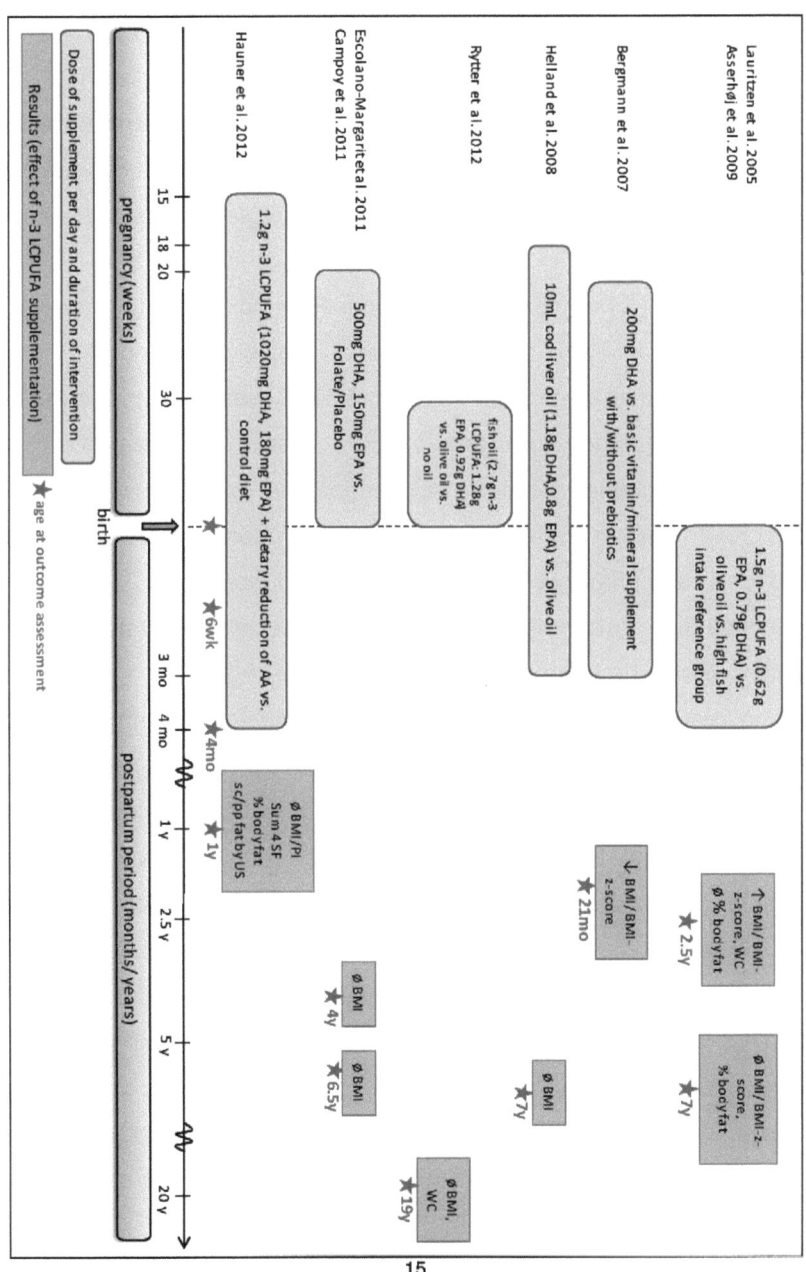

2   AIMS OF THE THESIS

Increasing awareness for the perinatal period as an important, sensitive phase for the programming of later disease susceptibility has stimulated research to develop innovative prevention strategies against childhood obesity.

The INFAT trial ("The *I*mpact of *N*utritional *F*atty acids during pregnancy and lactation for early human *A*dipose *T*issue development") was designed as a proof-of-concept study to test the hypothesis that lowering the n-6/n-3 long-chain fatty acid ratio in the diet of pregnant/breastfeeding women may reduce the expansion of adipose tissue growth early in life and may, thereby, represent a completely novel approach for the primary prevention of childhood obesity.

The intervention started early in pregnancy close to the first appearance of adipocytes in the human fetus (**Figure 2**) and lasted until 4 months of lactation, resulting in a broad time window of intervention during perinatal development.

In total, 208 women before their 15th week of gestation were enrolled and randomly assigned either to an intervention or a control group from the 15th week of pregnancy until 4 months postpartum. Primary outcome was infant fat mass estimated by skinfold thickness (SFT) measurements up to 12 months postpartum. Secondary endpoints included the fatty acid pattern of maternal blood, cord blood and breast milk, birth outcome (e.g., pregnancy duration), child growth and the sonographic assessment of abdominal subcutaneous and preperitoneal fat. The present work demonstrates the final analyses of the INFAT-study. The aims of the thesis were:

I) To study the potential effects of n-3 LCPUFAs supplementation during gestation and lactation on birth outcome, offspring growth and body composition up to 1 y of age

II) To study the potential association between a) maternal and b) cord blood n-3 LCPUFAs profile and infant growth and body composition

III) To study the potential association between breast milk n-3 LCPUFAs profile and infant growth and body composition

IV) To explore ultrasonography as a new body composition technique in infants ≤ 1 year of age and to cross-validate this method with anthropometry and SFT measurements

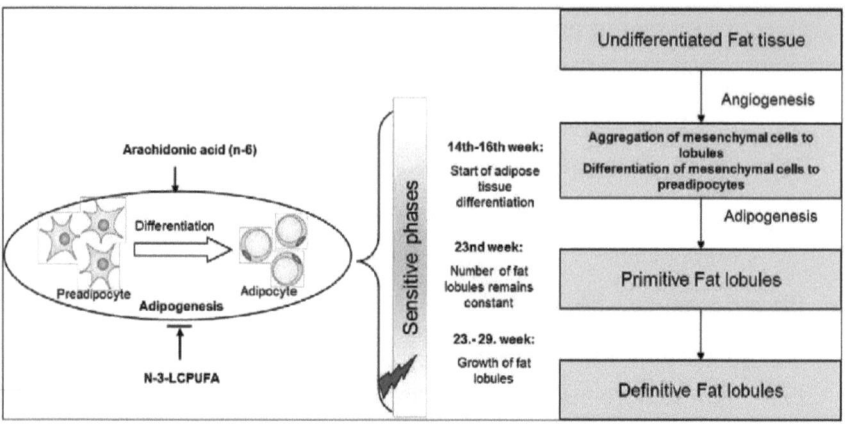

Figure 2: Sensitive phases of adipose tissue development and possible impact of LCPUFAs.

The first traces of fat cell development can be found between the 14th and 16th week of pregnancy. The morphogenesis of fat cell development is a continuous process with merging phases: In the first instance mesenchymal cell aggregates appear, which then form up specific tissue lobules. At the same time the formation of cappilaries begins and primitive and later on definitive fat lobules appear. The number of lobules remains constant from 23nd wk of gestation, whereas their size further increases up to 29th week of gestation (modified after Brunner et al. 2011 and Poissonnet et al. 1984). Thus, the period from 14th week of pregnancy onwards may constitute a sensitive phase for external influencing factors, e.g. the fatty acid composition of the maternal diet, which then might impact later obesity risk.

3 SUBJECTS AND METHODS

Many details of the subjects and methods applied have been published in Paper I (Hauner et al. 2012). The analysis of fatty acids was described in Paper II and III.

3.1 Study design

The INFAT study is an open-label, monocenter, prospective, randomized, controlled dietary intervention trial in a 2-arm parallel group design (Hauner et al. 2009). The study design is shown in **Figure 3**.

3.2 Recruitment

Between 14 July 2006 and 22 May 2009, healthy pregnant women before the 15th wk of gestation were recruited by 23 practice-based gynecologists in the Munich area, Germany, or directly by a research assistant in the outpatient clinic of the Division of Obstetrics and Perinatal Medicine of the University Hospital Klinikum rechts der Isar, Technische Universität München, Munich, Germany.

The study was also advertised in local newspapers, pregnancy specific Internet pages, and in a journal about pregnancy and baby care that is distributed monthly in pharmacies. The first screening was usually done by telephone or directly at the outpatient clinic by using a structured checklist.

3.3 Inclusion and exclusion criteria

Women who met the following inclusion criteria were enrolled: gestational age ≤15th wk of gestation, between 18 and 43 y of age, prepregnancy BMI (in kg/m^2) between 18 and 30, willingness to implement the dietary recommendations, sufficient German language skills, and written informed consent.

Exclusion criteria were as follows: high-risk pregnancy (multiple pregnancy, rhesus incompatibility, hepatitis B infection, or parity ≥ 4); hypertension (> 140/90 mm Hg); chronic diseases (eg, diabetes) or gastrointestinal disorders accompanied by maldigestion, malabsorption, or elevated energy and nutritional requirements (eg, gluten enteropathy); known metabolic defects (eg, phenylketonuria); psychiatric diseases; hyperemesis gravidarum; supplementation with n–3 LCPUFAs before randomization; and alcohol abuse and smoking.

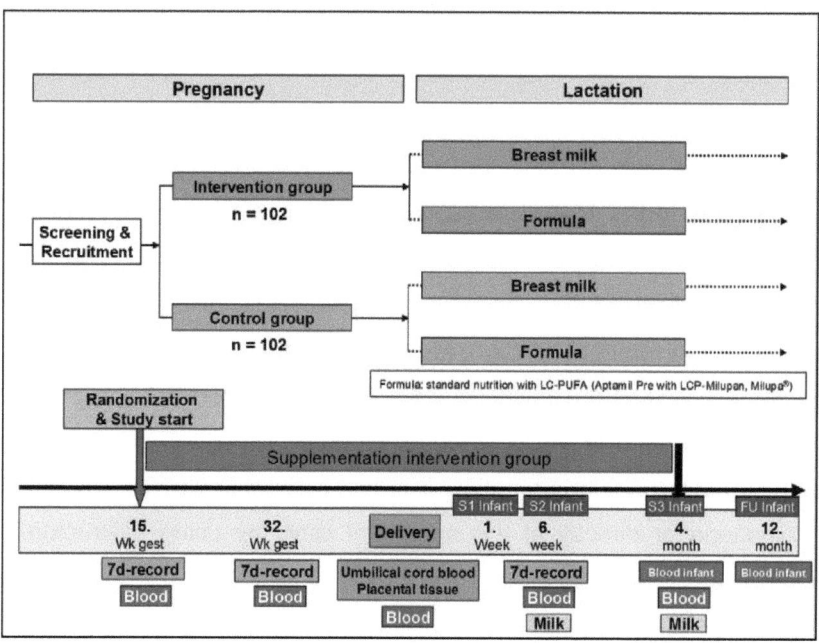

Figure 3: Study design

3.4 Screening examination

Women considered eligible for the study came to the study center (Else Kröner-Fresenius-Center for Nutritional Medicine, Klinikum rechts der Isar) before the 15th wk of gestation for the screening examination.

After detailed assessment of the medical history and filling in a questionnaire about lifestyle habits, current body height and weight, blood pressure, and the para/gravida status were retrieved from the maternity card.

3.5 Randomization, data management, and ethical requirements

Having obtained written informed consent from participants, randomization was performed in the 14th–15th wk of gestation by a research assistant.

Participants were randomly assigned on the basis of a computer-generated randomization sequence provided by the Institute for Medical Statistics and Epidemiology, Klinikum rechts der Isar, with 1:1 allocation in blocks to ensure balanced group sample sizes (SAS software version 9.1; SAS Institute Inc). All data from participants were collected by using case-report forms and were saved in an Access database (version 2003; Microsoft Corp). The study protocol was in accordance with the rules of the International Conference on Harmonization Good Clinical Practice guidelines (valid from 17 January 1997), the last revision of the declaration of Helsinki (October 2000; Edinburgh, United Kingdom), and applicable local regulatory requirements and laws. The study protocol was registered at clinicaltrials.gov as NCT00362089. The study protocol was approved by the ethical committee of the Technische Universität München (1479/06/2006/2/21).

3.6 Study groups and intervention

In total, 208 healthy pregnant women were randomly assigned either to the dietary intervention (n = 104) or control group (n = 104) from the 15th wk of gestation to 4 mo postpartum.

The intervention protocol combined 2 elements to reduce the ratio of n-6 to n-3 LCPUFAs from 7:1, which is the mean ratio in the German diet (Max-Rubner-Institut 2008) to a range of 3–3.5:1. Women received a fish oil supplement as 3 soft gel capsules (Marinol D-40; Lipid Nutrition) that contained in total 1200 mg n-3 LCPUFAs (1020 mg DHA and 180 mg EPA) as well as 9 mg vitamin E as an antioxidant per day during pregnancy and lactation. Simultaneously, the women received detailed nutritional counseling from trained research assistants. The women were asked to normalize the consumption of AA, which is an n-6 LCPUFAs that is mostly abundant in meat products and eggs, to a moderate amount of intake (~90 mg AA/d) compared with intakes from typical Western diets (~100–170 mg AA/d) (Kris-Etherton et al. 2000; Adam et al. 2003).

Dietary instructions to reduce AA intakes were based on a previous intervention study in patients with rheumatoid arthritis (Adam et al. 2003). The women were advised to replace AA-rich foods with foods low in AA and to limit their meat intake to 500 g/wk. Written information on the AA content of common foods was provided.

Participants of the control group received brief semi-structured counseling on a healthy balanced diet according to the guidelines of the German Nutrition Society (DGE) (Deutsche Gesellschaft für Ernährung e.V.) and were explicitly asked to refrain from taking fish oil or DHA supplements (Haffner et al. 1987).

3.7 Adverse events

All adverse events reported by the participating women were regularly assessed during visits and carefully documented.

3.8 Dietary intake

Dietary intake was assessed by 7-d dietary records completed by participants at the 15th (baseline) and 32nd wk of gestation and at 6 wk postpartum.

Trained research assistants carefully explained how to complete the dietary record and asked the women to estimate consumed foods in amounts usually used in the household (eg, one tablespoon or one cup).

Specific information on all sources of fat, including types of fish, seafood, meat, and meat products, was collected. Energy and macronutrient intakes and the consumption of specific fatty acids (AA, DHA, and EPA) were calculated with the nutrition software Prodi expert (version 5.3; Wissenschaftliche Verlagsgesellschaft mbH).

3.9 Blood and breast milk sampling

After an overnight fast, a ~30-mL venous blood sample was obtained from each participant at baseline (15th wk of gestation), 32nd wk of gestation, and 6 wk and 4 mo postpartum (if the mother was breastfeeding) to assess coagulation variables, blood glucose and lipids, and the maternal fatty acid profile in plasma and RBCs.

Cord blood was sampled from the umbilical vein at delivery. Maternal fasting breast milk samples were collected by breast pump (Medela Symphony; Eching, Germany) at 6 weeks pp and 4 months pp if mothers were breastfeeding their infant.

The time range between milk sample collection and the last breastfeeding was documented. Infant blood was collected by a pediatrician by venipuncture at 4 months and 12 months pp in a subsample, after parents gave written informed consent.

3.10 Fatty acid analysis in plasma phospholipids (PLs), red blood cells (RBCs) and breast milk

Venous blood samples were collected from each subject after fasting overnight in EDTA containing tubes and immediately centrifuged at 2000 x g for 10 minutes to separate erythrocytes and plasma. The plasma was removed and stored until analysis at $-86°C$. The erythrocytes were washed three times with 0.9% NaCl solution, aliquotted and stored until analysis at $-86°C$. The analysis of fatty acids was performed in the Laboratory of Lipid Research, Danone Research - Centre for Specialised Nutrition, Friedrichsdorf, Germany.

Extraction and separation of plasma lipids: Frozen plasma was thawed at room temperature and total lipids were extracted (with chloroform/methanol/water) according to the method of Bligh and Dyer (1959) (Bligh and Dyer 1959).The lipid classes were then separated by high performance liquid chromatography (HPLC) and fractionated via automatic fraction collection following a procedure described before (Beermann et al. 2005). The lipid class separation was performed with an HPLC Alliance 2695 Separation module from Waters (Waters GmbH, Eschborn, Germany) coupled to a PL-ELS 2100 evaporative light scattering detection system (Polymer Laboratories, Darmstadt, Germany). For lipid class separation, a PVA Sil column (5 μm, 250 mm x 8 mm) (YMC Europe, Dinslaken, Germany) was used. The eluent system corresponded to that of Christie (Christie and Urwin 1995).

Fatty acid derivatization: The separated PLs fraction of the HPLC fractionation was evaporated to dryness with nitrogen. Frozen erythrocytes and frozen milk were thawed at room temperature and directly applied to derivatization. For derivatization, the plasma PLs, the RBCs and breast milk samples were dissolved in 2 mL methanol/hexane (4:1, vol/vol) plus 0.5% pyrogallol as antioxidant, and were methylated according to Lepage and Roy (1984) (Lepage and Roy 1984) with 200 µL acetylchloride at 100°C, for 1h. Then 5 mL 6 % K_2CO_3 were added and the sample mixture was centrifuged for 10 min at 4°C with 3200 rpm. The upper hexane phase containing the fatty acid methyl esters (FAME) was then applied to further analysis.

Fatty acid methyl ester analysis: The FAME was analyzed by capillary gas chromatography (CGC) using a 6890N gas chromatograph (Agilent Technologies, Waldbronn, Germany) fitted with a cold-on-column injector (Beermann et al. 2005). A DB23 column (60 m, I.D. 0.25 mm, film 0.25 µm, JW Scientific, Agilent Technologies, US) was used for the separation of fatty acids. The chromatographic conditions were as follows: Injector (COC): 60 °C to 300 °C; carrier gas: hydrogen at a flow of 1,8 mL/min; flame ionization detector at 280 °C. Fatty acids were identified according to their retention times relative to standards (GLC 85 standard mix, NuChekPrep, Inc. Elysian, Minnesota, US). The CGC temperature program was as follows: initial temperature 60 °C for 0.1 min; from 60 °C to 160 °C at 40 °C/min; 160 °C for 2 min; from 160 °C to 190 °C at 3 °C/min; 190 °C to 220 °C at 4,5 °C/min, 220 °C for 5 min; from 220 °C to 240 °C at 5 °C/min; 240 °C for 25 min. Fatty acid values are presented in % FA/ total FA (% FA of total FA). All analyses were done in duplicate.

3.11 Compliance

The compliance of women with consumption of the fish-oil capsules was determined by repeated DHA and EPA analysis in RBCs, plasma PLs and breast milk lipids of the mothers and self-reported capsule-intake counting.

Women had to document the first ($\leq 15^{th}$ wk of gestation) and the last day the supplement was taken (≤ 4 mo postpartum) and the number of capsules ingested daily. If participants stopped breastfeeding before 4 mo postpartum, they had to stop the intake and to document the date. If the intake was missed, women had to record the reason why they did not take the supplement.

Capsule diaries were regularly checked for plausibility by a member of the study team. Capsules not taken had to be preserved and were counted at the next study visit. The compliance with DHA and EPA intakes was calculated by taking the number of fish-oil capsules ingested by the woman divided by the number the woman should have ingested and multiplied by 100. Women's compliance with the AA-balanced diet was assessed by 7-d dietary records (AA intake in mg/d).

The ratio of n-6/ n-3 PUFA from dietary intake was calculated by dividing the sum of the major n-6 PUFAs (linoleic acid and AA) by the sum of the major n-3 PUFAs (alpha-linolenic acid, EPA, and DHA) plus 1200 mg n-3 LCPUFAs intake from fish-oil capsules in the intervention group.

To support the intake of fish-oil capsules and to maintain compliance for the low-AA diet in the intervention group, the women were called every 4–8 wk by a member of the study team in addition to having regular study visits.

3.12 Infant growth and development

Birth weight and length, head circumference, sex of the newborn, and birth outcomes were collected from maternal obstetric records obtained from midwives of the obstetric clinics. At visit 6 wk and 4 and 12 mo postpartum, the weight of the naked infant was measured at the study center to the nearest 10 g with a standard infant scale (Babywaage Ultra MBSC-55; myweight). Height was measured with a measuring stick (Säuglingsmessstab seca 207; seca) to the nearest 0.5 cm while the infant was supine with stretched legs. Weight-for-length (in g/cm), BMI, (in kg/m^2) and the Ponderal index (in kg/m^3) were calculated from these measured variables.

3.13 Infant fat mass and fat distribution assessed by SFT

The SFT of the infant was the primary outcome variable. Longitudinal SFT measurements were performed by trained research-assistants 3–5 d postpartum in the obstetric clinic or at the family's home as well as at 6 wk postpartum and 4 and 12 mo postpartum at the study center (**Figure 4**).

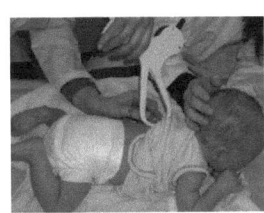
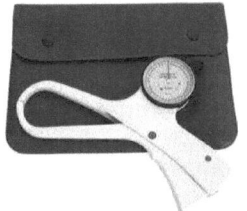

Figure 4: SFT measurement at 6 weeks pp   **Figure 5:** Holtain Caliper

The prespecified time point of primary interest was 4 mo postpartum, which reflected the termination of the dietary intervention. Reassessment at 12 mo was performed to detect long-term effects of the intervention.

SFTs were measured in triplicate under standard conditions with a Holtain caliper (Holtain Ltd, **Figure 5**) at the left body axis at the following 4 sites: 1) triceps, halfway between the acromion process and the olecranon process, 2) biceps, 2 cm proximal to the skin crease of the elbow, 3) subscapular, below the inferior angle of the left scapular and diagonal to the natural cleavage of the skin; and 4) suprailiac, along the midaxillary line above the iliac crest. The mean of the triplicate measurements was used for analysis.

The calculation of body fat (percentage) was done via predictive SFT equations according to the method of Weststrate and Deurenberg (Weststrate and Deurenberg 1989). To describe regional differences in subcutaneous body fat distribution, we calculated the sum of the 4 SFTs (sum of 4 SFT: biceps + triceps + subscapular + suprailiac) and the following 2 indexes of fat patterning: 1) the subscapular-to-triceps SFT ratio according to Haffner et al (Haffner et al. 1987) as an index of central to peripheral fat distribution and 2) the central-to-total SFT ratio (percentage of trunk-to-total SFTs) after Weststrate et al (Weststrate et al. 1989) by using the equation (Subscapular + suprailiac) : (sum of 4 SFTs) x 100.

3.14 Infant fat mass and fat distribution assessed by ultrasonography

To complement the primary endpoint with another method, ultrasonography was performed by 2 well-trained pediatricians who were blinded to group allocation (**Figure 6**). Abdominal subcutaneous fat and preperitoneal fat thickness, the latter of which is considered to be an approximation of visceral and intra-abdominal fat (Holzhauer et al. 2009), were measured longitudinally as areas of 1-cm length just below the xiphoid process at 6 wk and 4 and 12 mo postpartum, by using a high-resolution ultrasonographic system (Siemens Acuson Premium; Siemens) with a 10-MHz linear probe (VFX 13–5; Siemens Medical Solutions, **Figure 7**).

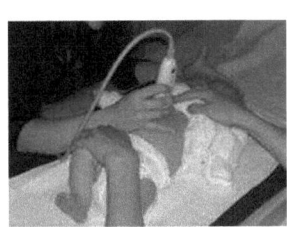

Figure 6: Sonographic investigation at 6 weeks pp

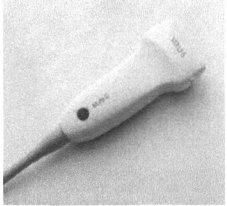

Figure 7: 10-MHz linear probe

The technique used was a modification of the method recently described by Holzhauer et al (Holzhauer et al. 2009). Subcutaneous fat was determined in sagittal (**Figure 8 and 9**) and axial planes (**Figure 10 and 11**) in the middle of the xiphoid process and the navel directly above the linea alba.

Subjects and methods

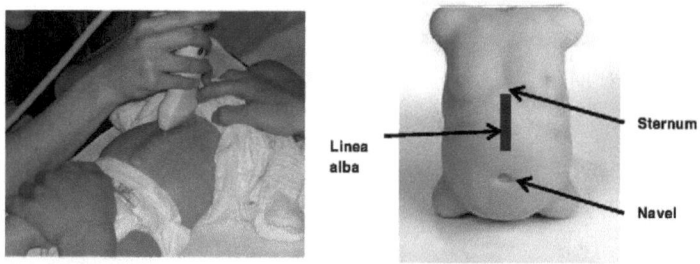

Figure 8: Sonographic assessment in **sagittal** direction. Right schematic picture: the blue line labels the direction of the linear probe.

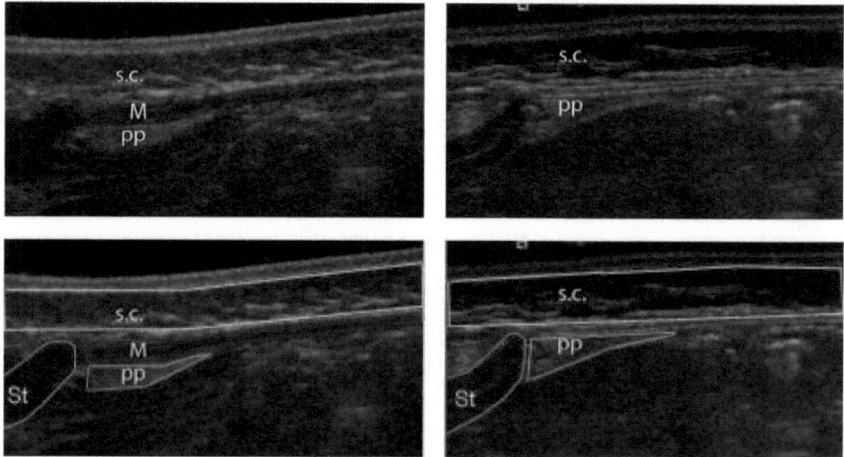

Figure 9: Examples for demonstration of the holding technique in **sagittal** plane.

Left pictures, colored lines: Picture next to the linea alba and therefore out of measurement area, demonstrated by muscle in the picture, which is echo-poor (M, blue), therefore reduced preperitoneal fat layer (pp, orange); the thickness of subcutaneous fat remains unaffected (s.c.,yellow).

Right pictures: Correct holding technique in the measurement area. Direction of the linear probe exactly along the linea alba, demonstrated by lack of muscle tissue. s.c.: subcutaneous yellow; pp: preperitoneal, orange. St: Sternum, green.

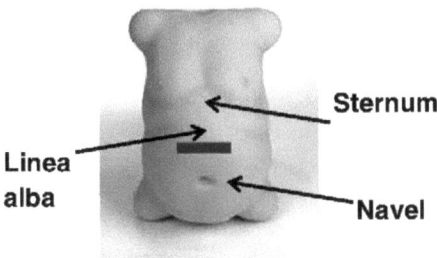

Figure 10: Sonographic assessment in axial direction; schematic picture: the blue line demonstrates the direction of the linear probe

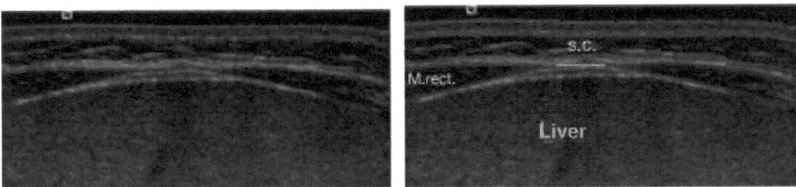

Figure 11: Examples for the holding technique in the **axial** plane.

Right picture with colored labeling of the anatomic structures; yellow: linea alba; s.c.: subcutaneous (red); M.rect.= Musculus rectus abdominis (blue)

We did not only measure the thickness of SC fat as distance between upper and lower border of the respective fat layer, but introduced areas of preperitoneal and subcutaneous fat as a measure of thickness of fat layers according to Holzhauer and colleagues to optimize precision and accuracy of the method and to allow for age specific differences in anatomy (Holzhauer et al. 2009).

Analysis of the ultrasound images was performed in a strictly blinded fashion. The ratio of subcutaneous to preperitoneal fat was calculated by using the mean of subcutaneous sagittal and axial fat layers divided by the area of preperitoneal fat (subcutaneous:preperitoneal ratio).

3.15 Evaluation of the ultrasound images

The size of the individual fat layers was determined with Osirix software (http://www.osirix-viewer.com, Genf, Schweiz) in the sagittal and axial plane.

Preperitoneal fat

The preperitoneal fat layer was evaluated in sagittal plane, only.

Preperitoneal fat was defined as distance between the linea alba as the upper border and the peritoneum located at the upper margin of the liver as the lower border. The first measurement was performed 0.5 cm caudal from the xiphoid process (sag_i cranial pp) while the second measurement was performed 1 cm caudal from the first reference point (sag_i caudal pp) (**Figure 12**).

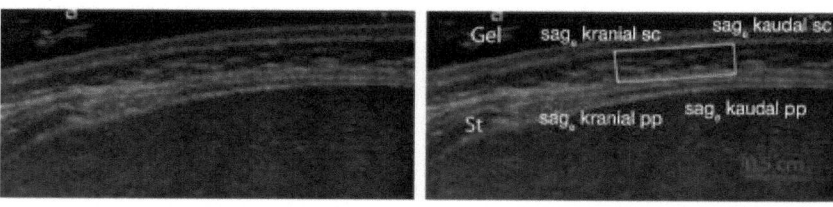

Figure 12: Example for measurements in the sagittal plane with labeling of the measurement area in subcutaneous fat (yellow) and preperitoneal fat (orange) and labeling of the reference points sag_i cranial sc and sag_i caudal sc as well as sag_i cranial pp and sag_i caudal pp in the right picture; St = Sternum; red: scale 0.5 cm at the right lower border of the picture.

The mean was calculated from 3 images (sag cranial pp, sag caudal pp). The area of preperitonal fat was calculated following the formula for trapezoid areas.

$$Asag\,pp = \frac{sag\,cranial\,pp[cm] + sag\,caudal\,pp[cm]}{2} \times 1[cm]$$

In case of strong bending the area of preperitoneal fat was calculated by approximation by the help of two trapezoids.

Subcutaneous fat

The subcutaneous fat was defined as the echo-poor space between the echo-rich cutis and the echo-rich linea alba (M. rectus abdominis). The subcutaneous fat layer was determined in both, the sagittal and axial plane.

In axial plane the measurement was performed directly above the linea alba (ax_i m) as well as 1cm on the right (ax_i r) and left (ax_i l) of the linea alba between the M. rectus abdominis and the cutis (**Figure 13**).

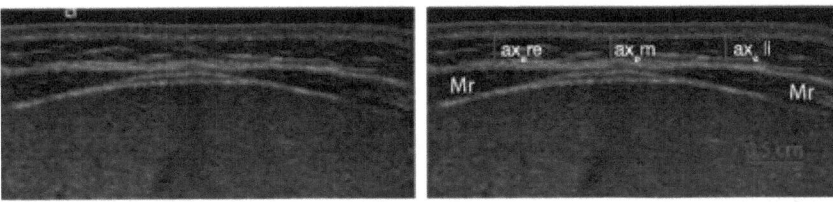

Figure 13: Example of a measurement in the axial plane (down) with labeling of the measurement area in subcutaneous fat layer (red) as well as the reference points ax_i r, ax_i m and ax_i l in the right picture; Mr: M. rectus abdominis.

In sagittal plane the first reference point was set 1 cm caudal the xyphoid process, the lower margin of the sternum (sag_i cranial sc) and the second reference point 1cm caudal of the first reference point (sag_i caudal sc), to take advantage of the space where the layers exert highest parallelism. The measurements were repeated in all 3 images and the mean was calculated out of these measures (sag cranial sc, sag caudal sc, ax r, ax m, ax l).

The sagittal area was calculated following the pictured formula:

$$A sag sc = \frac{sag cranial sc [cm] + sag caudal sc [cm]}{2} \times 1[cm].$$

For the axial area the mean of all subcutaneous layers was calculated.

$$A ax sc = \left(\frac{axr[cm] + axl[cm]}{2} \times 1[cm] + \frac{axm[cm] + axl[cm]}{2} \times 1[cm] \right) \bigg/ 2$$

Moreover, the ratio of subcutaneous and preperitoneal fat tissue was calculated.

$$R sc / pp = \frac{\frac{A sag sc + A ax sc}{2}}{A sag pp}$$

In general the fat layers showed very heterogenous structures in the infants investigated (**Figure 14, 15, 16**).

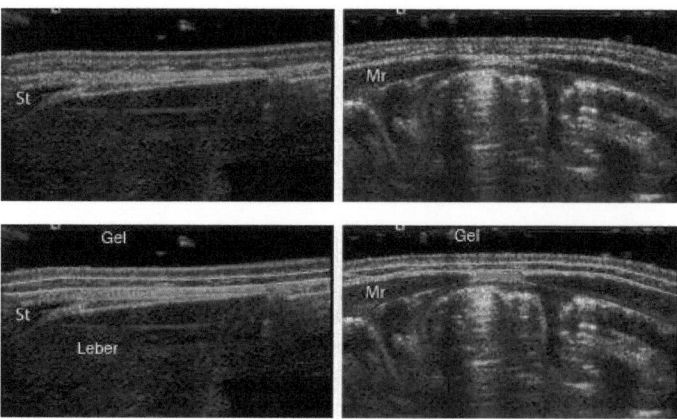

Figure 14: Thin subcutaneous fat layer

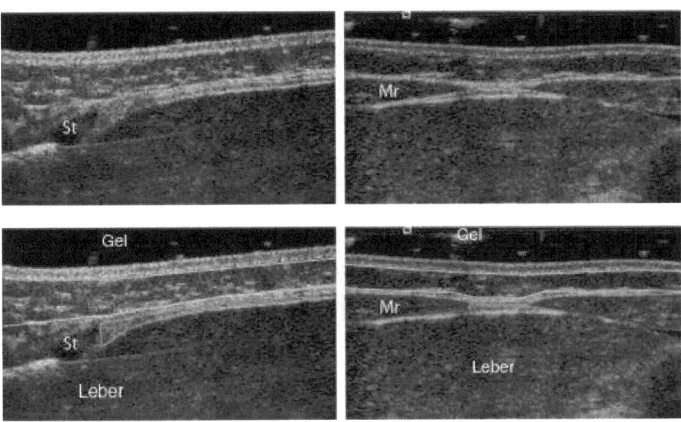

Figure 15: Medium thickness of subcutaneous fat layer

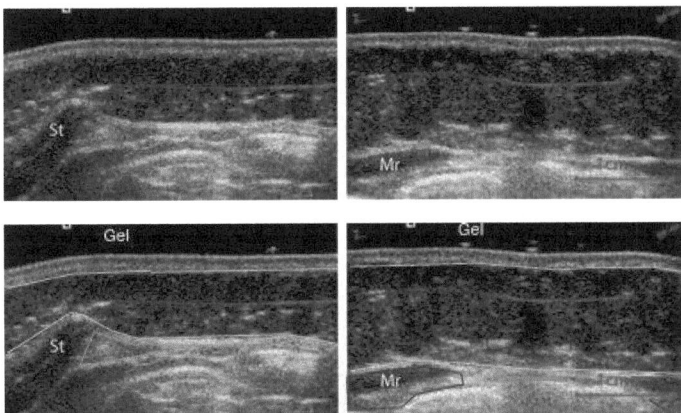

Figure 16: Large thickness of subcutaneous fat layer

Figure 14, Figure 15, Figure 16: Figures showing different thicknesses of subcutaneous (yellow) fat tissue; images in the **sagittal** plane are shown on the left and images in the **axial** plane are shown on the right; the colored figures demonstrate the anatomic structure. Mr: Musculus rectus abdominis, St: Sternum; Colored Lines: yellow: subcutaneous adipose tissue; orange: preperitoneal fat; blue: Musculus rectus abdominis; green: Linea alba

3.16 Blinding of participants and study team

The specific intervention of the INFAT study did not allow a double-blind design; however, to avoid bias, the number of visits and dietary counseling was the same in both groups. Appointments for dietary counseling were scheduled individually with the women to avoid an exchange of information between groups.

The research staff who assessed the SFT (primary endpoint) and infant growth was not blinded to study-group allocation. In contrast, the ultrasound measurements were performed by trained pediatricians who were strictly blinded to group allocation and explicitly not involved in any other aspects of the study.

3.17 Statistical analysis

With the minimum sample size of 104 patients per group, the study had a power of 80% to detect effect sizes ≤ 0.5 (Cohen's d) in the sum of the 4 defined SFTs at 4 mo postpartum between study groups with a type I error level of 0.05 (2-sided).

This relative effect size translated to detectable differences in SFT from 2.5 to ≤5 mm (ie, the sum of 4 SFTs), considering expected standard deviations from 5 mm (Schmelzle and Fusch 2002) up to a conservatively assumed maximum of 10 mm. The chosen effect size of 0.5 was further defined as the medium effect size, which reflects the consideration to not investigate too small (clinically irrelevant) or too big (overly optimistic) effect sizes. The sample-size calculation took into account a dropout rate of 30%. Analyses were based on all women who were randomly assigned by following an intention-to-treat approach.

Discrete variables are shown as numbers (percentages) and were compared by using chi-square analysis. Continuous variables are presented as means ± SDs and were tested by using the Mann-Whitney U test. Bonferroni correction of P values was applied to reduce multiple test issues within the secondary analysis. Group differences in maternal birth outcomes and complications were assessed by risk ratios with 95% CIs.

For analyses of the primary outcome (ie, the sum of 4 SFTs) and secondary outcomes, mean differences and 95% CIs were calculated. Changes in maternal fatty acid profile over time were determined by using the Friedman-Test or Wilkoxon-Test. To determine the relationship between 1) maternal and cord blood RBCs and infant outcomes and 2) breast milk fatty acids and infant outcomes, the Spearman-Rho correlation coefficient was calculated based on the entire study population, in addition to linear regression models. Because the main neonatal outcomes were strongly affected by the duration of pregnancy, multiple linear regression models (F test and ANCOVA) and partial correlations were used in the analysis of infant growth and infant fat mass to correct for effects mediated by this and other relevant confounders. Intra- and inter-observer agreements of sonographic measurements were examined using intraclass correlation coefficients (ICC) and their 95% confidence intervals. An ICC of 1 indicates that all of the observed variation is caused by between subject variations. Statistical analyses were performed with the R software package (version 2.8.1; R Foundation for Statistical Computing) and PASW software (version 17.0; SPSS Inc).

4 RESULTS

4.1 Clinical data and comparison of the randomized groups

The results of the clinical data analysis have been published in Paper I (Hauner et al. 2012).

4.1.1 Participant characteristics

A total of 208 women were included in the study before the 15th wk of gestation. The study population was of Causcasian origin (except for one Asian woman), relatively well-educated, nonsmoking, with an average age of 32 y, and had a mean prepregnancy BMI of 22 (**Table 1**).

Maternal clinical characteristics, maternal diet and lifestyle factors, and socio-demographic variables of the 2 groups were comparable at baseline (Table 1). We analyzed 188 newborns (90.4%), 185 infants at 3–5 d postpartum (88.9%), 180 infants at 6 wk postpartum (86.5%), 174 infants at 4 mo postpartum (83.7%), and 170 1-y olds (81.7%). The last baby was born in November 2010. Reasons for the loss to the follow-up examination at 1 y are shown in **Figure 17**.

4.1.2 Compliance

The compliance of women with the fish-oil intake and the AA-balanced diet is illustrated in **Table 2**.

Overall, 96.3% (n = 86) of women in the intervention group took ≥ 90% of the capsules. Two women (2.2%) ingested ≥ 80% to ≤ 90% of the capsules. One woman (1.1%) took only 72% of the supplements. Main reasons for leftover capsules were gastrointestinal disorder because of virus infection, vacation, or postpartum hospital stay. Compliance was further confirmed by measurements of the fatty acid profile in maternal RBCs.

The fatty acid composition of RBCs was comparable in the 2 groups at study entry (Table 2). The intervention resulted in a substantial increase in the relative content of DHA and EPA in maternal RBCs at week 32 of gestation and a modest decrease in AA associated with a remarkable, significant decrease of the n-6/n-3 LCPUFAs ratio (P< 0.001) in the intervention group compared with in the control group, which further assured compliance to the intervention.

The maternal dietary intake of AA (in mg/d and mg/1000 kcal) differed significantly between groups at the 32nd wk of pregnancy (Table 2). AA consumption was lower in the intervention group than in the control group (129.8 ± 76.6 compared with 160.6 ± 80.6 mg/d and 62.8 6 34 compared with 78.7 ± 42.9 mg/1000 kcal, respectively; P < 0.01). Thus, at week 32 of gestation, the dietary n-6/n-3 PUFA ratio was ~3.5:1 in the intervention group compared with ~7:1 in the control group, as originally intended (Table 2).

Table 1: Characteristics of the study population at baseline[1]

	Intervention group (n=104)	Control group (n=103[2])
Mean (± SD)		
Age [years]	31.9 (± 4.9)	31.6 (± 4.5)
Weight before pregnancy [kg]	63.9 (± 9.2)	63.2 (± 8.4)
Height [cm]	169.2 (± 6.5)	168.1 (± 5.3)
BMI before pregnancy [kg/m²]	22.3 (± 2.9)	22.4 (± 3.0)
Gestational age [weeks]	14.6 (± 1.2)	14.5 (± 1.1)
Weight at study entry [kg]	66.2 (± 9.7)	65.6 (± 8.3)
Blood pressure systolic [mm/Hg]	113.6 (± 13.1)	112.4 (± 10.3)
Blood pressure diastolic [mm/Hg]	69.6 (± 8.4)	68.5 (± 8.8)
% of the group		
Attended ≥ 12 years at school	63.8	69.9
Primiparae	55.8	61.2
Smoking before pregnancy	16.3	24.3
Alcohol before pregnancy	65.4	65.0
during pregnancy	2.9	4.9
Specific diet during pregnancy		
no	92.9	95.0
vegetarian	2.0	2.0
vegetarian+ fish	2.0	2.0
lactose free	3.1	0
other diets	0	1.0

[1] Values are shown as mean ± SD (n) or percentage of the group (n). For quantitative variables the Mann-Whitney-test was used (p< 0.05); for qualitative variables, the Chi-Square test was used (p< 0.05). There were no significant differences between the intervention and the control group at baseline (15th week of gestation).

[2] One woman of the control group dropped out, before the complete baseline data could be assessed

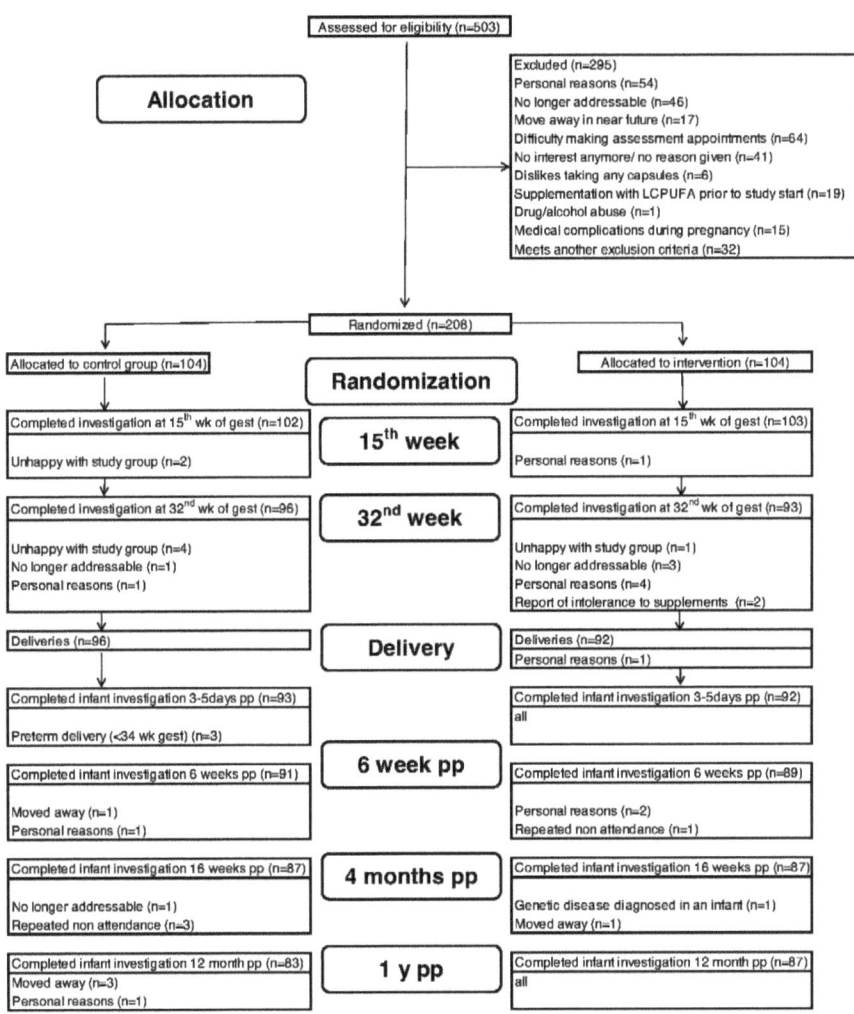

Figure 17: Flow Chart of the INFAT-study

Table 2: Women's compliance with the fish oil intake and the AA-balanced diet[1]

		Intervention group	Control group
		% of the group (n)	% of the group (n)
Women's intake of fish oil capsules			
< 80%		1.1% (1)	-
≥ 80% and < 90%		2.2% (2)	-
≥ 90%		96.6% (86)	-
Dietary intake at 32nd wk of gest		% or mean ± SD (n)	
Energy [kcal/day]		2052 ± 379 (83)	2106 ± 449 (83)
Protein [%]		14.8% (83)	14.7% (83)
Fat [%]		32.7% (83)	33.8% (83)
Carbohydrates [%]		52.3% (83)	51.2% (83)
Linoleic acid [g/day]		9.7 ± 3.3 (83)	10.0 ± 4.1 (83)
Alpha-linolenic acid [g/day]		1.3 ± 0.5 (83)	1.3 ± 0.6 (83)
Eicosapentaenoic acid [mg/day]		111 ± 223.5 (83)	88.0 ± 135.5 (83)
Docosahexaenoic acid [mg/day]		201.2 ± 258.3 (83)	198.8 ± 220.1 (83)
Arachidonic acid [mg/day]		129.8 ± 76.6 (83)**	160.6 ± 80.6 (83)
Arachidonic acid [mg/1000 kcal]		62.8 ± 34 (83)**	78.7 ± 42.9 (83)
n-6/n-3 PUFA ratio [2]		3.5 ± 1.2 (83)***	6.9 ± 3.3 (83)
Maternal fatty acid profile in RBCs		mean ± SD (n)	
Eicosapentaenoic acid (20:5n3)	15th wk	0.42 ± 0.18 (100)	0.42 ± 0.15 (102)
	32nd wk	0.66 ± 0.32 (93)***	0.33 ± 0.16 (92)
Docosahexaenoic acid (22:6n3)	15th wk	4.55 ± 1.61 (100)	4.54 ± 1.24 (102)
	32nd wk	7.18 ± 2.97 (93)***	4.34 ± 2.07 (95)
Arachidonic acid (20:4n6)	15th wk	11.83 ± 3.1 (102)	12.51 ± 2.3 (102)
	32nd wk	8.82 ± 2.84 (93)***	10.15 ± 3.89 (95)
n-6/n-3 LCPUFAs ratio [3]	15th wk	2.77 ± 1.03 (101)	2.70 ± 0.64 (102)
	32nd wk	1.54 ± 0.63 (91)***	2.80 ± 1.17 (95)

[1] Data are presented as mean ± SD (n) or percentage of the group (n). For quantitative variables the Mann-Whitney-test was used (p< 0.05); for qualitative variables, the Chi-Square test was used (p< 0.05). Values for fatty acids are expressed as % of total fatty acids (% FA).

Values marked with stars show significant differences between groups at 32nd week of gestation (Mann-Whitney-U-Test, **p ≤ 0.01; ***p ≤ 0.001) after Bonferroni-corrections

[2] n-6/n-3 PUFA ratio: (C18:2n6 + C20:4n6) / (C18:3n3 + C20:5n3 + C22:6n3 + (for intervention group only) 1200 mg n-3 LCPUFAs from supplement)

[3] n-6/n-3 LCPUFAs ratio: (C20:2n6 + C20:3n6 + C20:4n6 + C22:2n6 + C22:4n6 + C22:5n6) / (C20:3n3 + C20:4n3 + C20:5n3 + C21:5n3 + C22:3n3 + C22:5n3 + C22:6n3)

4.1.3 Blood coagulation and tolerance

Blood coagulation variables were similar in both groups (**Appendix 1**). No side effects of the intervention were observed (data not shown).

4.1.4 Pregnancy outcomes and complications

A total of 188 women from the INFAT study gave birth to healthy infants during the time period of February 2007 to November 2009.

Forty-eight percent of newborns were girls, and 52% of newborns were boys. As illustrated in **Table 3**, the average duration of gestation was prolonged in the intervention group compared with in the control group (280 ± 8.5 d compared with 275 ± 11.4 d; $P = 0.001$), with a mean difference of 4.8 d (95% CI: 1.19, 7.67) between groups.

However, all infants were born full term between 37th and 42nd wk of gestation except for 3 preterm infants in the intervention (3.3%), 4 preterm infants in the control group (4.2%), and one postterm baby in the intervention group (1.1%). Thus, there was no significant shift in the frequencies of preterm, term, and postterm deliveries between groups, toward an increased risk of postterm pregnancies in the intervention group [risk ratio: 3.13 (95% CI: 0.13, 75.84].

This result might be partly explained by a tendency toward a higher rate of induced deliveries at term within the intervention group (23.9%; n = 22) compared with in the control group (13.5%; n = 13) [risk ratio: 1.75 (95% CI: 0.94, 3.26)].

There were no significant differences in birth complications such as a prolonged process of labor, cessation of labor, excessive blood loss at delivery, or placenta retention (Table 3).

Table 3: Birth outcomes and complications[1]

	Intervention group (n=92)	Control group (n=96)	Mean difference or RR (95 % CI)
Mean ± SD (n)			
Pregnancy duration [days]	279.9 ± 8.5 (92)	275.1 ± 11.4 (96)	4.8 (1.91, 7.67)***
Gestational weight gain [kg] [2]	15.1 ± 4.8 (91)	16.0 ± 5.1 (95)	-0.9 (-2.32, 0.52)
Blood loss at delivery [ml]	377 ± 153 (92)	366 ± 124 (96)	11 (-29, 51)
APGAR-score	9.7 ± 0.5 (92)	9.6 ± 0.7 (95)	0.1 (-0.1, 0.3)
% of the group (n)			
Complications			
Gestational Diabetes mellitus [3]	7.6 (7)	10.4 (10)	0.73 (0.29, 1.84)
Pathological cardiotocography [4]	23.9 (22)	18.8 (18)	1.28 (0.73, 2.22)
Cessation of labour [4]	14.1 (13)	11.5 (11)	1.23 (0.58, 2.61)
Placental retention [4]	9.8 (9)	5.2 (5)	1.88 (0.65, 5.40)
Birth mode			
Spontaneous birth	52.2 (48)	56.3 (54)	0.93 (0.71, 1.21)
Caeserian Section	33.7 (31)	32.3 (31)	1.04 (0.69, 1.57)
Vacuum extraction	14.1 (13)	11.5 (11)	1.23 (0.58, 2.61)
Induction of labour	23.9 (22)	13.5 (13)	1.75 (0.94, 3.26)
Classification of the newborns [4]			
Preterm birth	3.3 (3)	4.2 (4)	0.78 (0.18, 3.40)
Term birth	95.7 (88)	95.8 (92)	1.00 (0.94, 1.06)
Postterm birth	1.1 (1)	0 (0)	3.13 (0.13, 75.84)
Large for gestational age (> 90. P)	9.8 (9)	7.3 (7)	1.34 (0.52, 3.45)
Breastfeeding status at 4 months			
Exclusively breastfed	65.9 (58)	62.9 (56)	1.05 (0.84, 1.30)
Formula and breast milk	12.5 (11)	18.0 (16)	0.70 (0.34, 1.14)
Formula only	21.6 (19)	19.1 (17)	1.13 (0.63, 2.03)

[1] Data are presented as mean ± SD (n) or percentage of the group (n). For quantitative variables the Student's t-test was used (p< 0.05); for qualitative variables, the Chi-Square test was used (p< 0.05). Values marked with stars show significant differences between groups (Student's t-test, ***p≤ 0.001).
[2] last measured value at booking minus self-reported weight before pregnancy
[3] defined according to the new diagnostic criteria of the Hypergycemia and adverse pregnancy outcome study (HAPO-study) (Coustan et al. 2010)
[4] defined according to the German Society for Gynecology and Obstetrics e.V. (German Society for Gynecology and Obstetrics eV.)

4.1.5 Infant growth

Growth patterns of infants from birth during the first year of life are presented in **Table 4** and **Figure 18**.

Lengths and head circumferences did not significantly differ between groups at any point in time, except at delivery, where newborns in the intervention group showed a higher birth weight than did newborns in the control group [3534 ± 465 g (n = 92) compared with 3357 ± 557 g (n = 96), respectively; difference: 178 g (95% CI: 31, 324); P = 0.019] and a higher weight-for-length, BMI, and Ponderal index than did newborns in control group (Table 4).

Greater weight and growth indexes at birth were caused by prolonged gestation in the intervention group, as indicated in a linear adjusted model; when the group difference in birth weight was corrected for pregnancy duration and sex, the difference between groups was not significant [47 g (95% CI: 281, 175; P = 0.473]. Differences in body weight and relative growth indexes at birth disappeared over the first year of life and were not detectable at 6 wk and 4 and 12 mo postpartum, respectively (Table 4).

Table 4: Growth pattern and growth indices from birth up to 1 year of life[1]

		Intervention group mean ± SD (n)	Control group mean ± SD (n)	Unadjusted mean difference (95 % CI)	Adjusted mean difference (95% CI)
Weight [g]	birth	3534 ± 465 (92)	3357 ± 557 (96)	178 (31, 324)*	47 (-81, 175)
	6 weeks	4793 ± 606 (89)	4736 ± 625 (91)	57 (-123, 237)	-15 (-188, 158)
	4 months	6476 ± 679 (87)	6303 ± 724 (87)	176 (-32, 208)	120 (-83, 323)
	12 months	9650 ± 1025 (87)	9379 ± 1035 (83)	271 (-39, 508)	198 (-97, 494)
Length [cm]	birth	51.9 ± 2.2 (92)	51.5 ± 2.8 (96)	0.4 (-0.3, 1.1)	-0.2 (-0.8, 0.5)
	6 weeks	56.0 ± 2.0 (89)	55.6 ± 2.6 (91)	0.4 (-0.3, 1.1)	0.1 (-0.5, 0.7)
	4 months	62.6 ± 2.0 (88)	62.4 ± 2.2 (87)	0.2 (-0.4, 120.8)	0.0 (-0.6, 0.6)
	12 months	75.5 ± 2.4 (87)	74.9 ± 2.8 (83)	0.7 (-0.1, 199.2)	0.6 (-0.2, 1.4)
BMI [kg/m²]	birth	13.1 ± 1.2 (92)	12.6 ± 1.3 (96)	0.5 (0.2, 0.9)**	0.3 (-0.1, 0.6)
	6 weeks	15.2 ± 1.4 (89)	15.3 ± 1.2 (91)	-0.0 (-0.4, 0.4)	-0.1 (-0., 0.3)
	4 months	16.5 ± 1.4 (87)	16.2 ± 1.3 (87)	0.3 (-0.1, 0.9)	0.3 (-0.1, 0.7)
	12 months	16.9 ± 1.5 (87)	16.7 ± 1.4 (83)	0.2 (-0.2, 0.4)	0.1 (-0.3, 0.5)
Head circumference [cm]	birth	35.1 ± 1.4 (92)	34.8 ± 1.7 (96)	0.3 (-0.2, 0.7)	-0.1 (-0.5, 0.3)
	6 weeks	38.4 ± 1.1 (89)	38.3 ± 1.2 (90)	0.1 (-0.3, 0.4)	-0.1 (-0.4, 0.2)
	4 months	41.2 ± 1.3 (87)	41.0 ± 1.3 (87)	0.2 (-0.2, 0.6)	0.1 (-0.3, 0.4)
	12 months	46.5 ± 1.6 (87)	46.1 ± 1.5 (83)	0.4 (-0.0, 0.9)	0.4 (-0.1, 0.8)
Weight/length [g/cm]	birth	67.9 ± 7.2 (92)	64.9 ± 8.5 (96)	3.1 (0.8, 5.3)**	1.1 (-0.9, 3.1)
Ponderal Index [kg/m³]	birth	25.2 ± 2.3 (92)	24.4 ± 2.4 (96)	0.8 (0.1, 1.5)*	0.5 (-0.2, 1.2)

[1] Data are presented as mean ± SD (n) along with the non-adjusted mean difference (95% confidence interval). Values marked with stars show significant differences between groups (Student's t-test, *p<0.05; **p<0.01). The last column gives the adjusted mean difference (95% CI) from multiple regression analysis (F-test, ANCOVA) controlling for sex and pregnancy duration in the analysis at birth, 6 weeks and 4 months and, additionally, for Ponderal Index at birth and breastfeeding status at 4 months in the analysis of the 1 year olds.

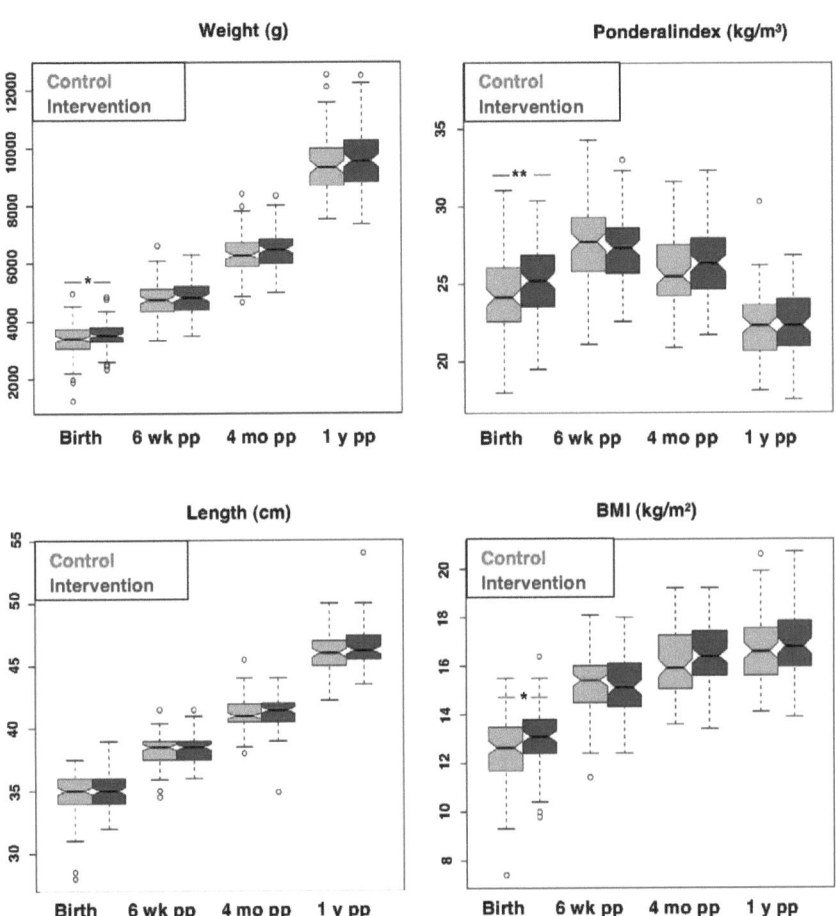

Figure 18: Growth pattern of the infants from birth up to 1 year of life. Data are presented as notched box-plots. Notched box-plots apply a "notch" or narrowing of the box around the median. Bottom and top edges of the box are located at 25th and 75th percentiles, center horizontal line is drawn at the median, whiskers mark the maximum and minimum. Outliners are shown as dots. Values marked with stars show significant differences between groups (Mann-Whitney-U-Test, *$p < 0.05$; **$p \leq 0.01$).

4.1.6 Infant fat mass and distribution

Fat-mass development and distribution assessed by SFT investigations are presented in **Table 5**.

Neither the 4 individual SFTs (**Figure 19**) nor their calculated sum differed (**Figure 20**) between groups at any of the 4 time points investigated.

At 4 mo postpartum, the sum of 4 SFTs was 25.3 ± 4.1 mm in the intervention group (n = 87) and 25.2 ± 4.3 mm (n = 87) in the control group [mean difference: 0.1 (95% CI: 21.2, 1.2)] in the uncorrected analysis. To consider observed group differences in pregnancy duration and consecutive higher birth weights, we performed multiple regression analyses. After adjustment for pregnancy duration (ie, the main confounder) and sex, the mean difference was not significantly different between groups at 4 mo postpartum (0.3 [95%: CI 21.0, 1.5]). During reassessment at age 1 y, unadjusted values were comparable between intervention and control groups [24.1 ± 4.4 mm (n = 85) compared with 24.1 ± 4.1 mm (n = 80); difference: 20.0 (95% CI: 21.3, 1.3)]. Similar results were obtained in the multiple regression model (Table 5) when variables of offspring fat mass were corrected for relevant confounders (eg, Ponderal index at birth, degree of breastfeeding at month 4 (ie, exclusive, partly, or formula), sex, and pregnancy duration) in the analysis of 1-y olds [sum of 4 SFTs at 12 mo: 24.1 ± 4.4 mm (n = 85) in the intervention group compared with 24.1 ± 4.1 mm (n = 80) in the control group; mean difference: 0.1 mm (21.2, 1.4 mm)]. Additional controlling for parity did not significantly affect the results of the primary endpoint to ≤1 y of age. Likewise, the percentage of body fat and body fat mass in grams as estimated by a predictive SFT equation were not significantly different between groups at 3–5 d, 6 wk, and 4 and 12 mo postpartum.

The subscapular-to-triceps ratio and the trunk-to-total SFT percentages did not show significant differences between intervention and control groups over the time course; thus, the pattern of adipose tissue distribution (central compared with peripheral) was comparable between groups.

Adipose tissue growth and abdominal fat distribution at 6 wk and 4 and 12 mo postpartum assessed by ultrasonography are shown in **Table 6**. We observed no significant differences between groups in any variable of fat mass determined by ultrasonography at the time points investigated, which corresponded to the results of SFT measurements. Adipose tissue development of both subcutaneous and preperitoneal areas had the same temporal pattern in intervention and control groups during the first year of life.

The fat distribution in the upper abdomen of the infants was also comparable between groups, as indicated by the subcutaneous:preperitoneal ratio (Table 6). At 1 y of age, the subcutaneous area was 30.7 ± 14.2 mm^2 in the intervention group (n = 79) compared with 32.3 ± 16.6 mm^2 in the control group (n = 77). The preperitoneal area was 17.6 ± 0.1 mm^2 in infants in the intervention group (n = 76) compared with 18.2 ± 0.1 mm^2 in infants in the control group (n = 77). The mean difference between groups was 21.6 mm^2 (95% CI: 26.4, 3.2 mm^2) in subcutaneous area and 20.6 mm^2 (95% CI: 22.4, 1.3 mm^2) in the preperitoneal area in favor of the intervention group, but this result was not significantly different even after adjustment for current weight and length (Table 6).

Table 5: Adipose tissue growth and subcutaneous fat distribution during the first year of life assessed by skinfold thickness measurements[1]

		Intervention group mean ± SD (n)	Control group mean ± SD (n)	Unadjusted mean difference (95 % CI)	Adjusted mean difference (95% CI)
Age [days] at SFT	3-5 d	4.7 ± 2.4 (84)	4.6 ± 2.1 (84)	0.1 (-0.6, 0.8)	
	6 wk	44.4 ± 6.2 (89)	44.5 ± 6.6 (91)	-0.2 (-2, 1.7)	
	4 mo	110.3 ± 6.9 (87)	110.6 ± 8.9 (87)	-0.2 (-2.6, 2.1)	
	12 mo	377.1 ± 16.2 (87)	378.6 ± 17.1 (83)	-1.6 (-6.6, 3.4)	
Sum of 4 SFT [mm]	3-5 d	16.1 ± 2.6 (84)	15.8 ± 2.7 (84)	0.3 (-0.5, 1.1)	0.3 (-0.5, 1.2)
	6 wk	21.9 ± 4.0 (89)	22.2 ± 3.5 (91)	-0.3 (-1.4, 0.8)	-0.4 (-1.5, 0.8)
	4 mo	25.3 ± 4.1 (87)	25.2 ± 4.3 (87)	0.1 (-1.2, 1.2)	0.3 (-1.0, 1.5)
	12 mo	24.1 ± 4.4 (85)	24.1 ± 4.1 (80)	-0.0 (-1.3, 1.3)	0.1 (-1.2, 1.4)
Fat mass [g]	3-5 d	501 ± 142 (84)	473 ± 142 (84)	29 (-15, 71)	20 (-24, 64)
	6 wk	916 ± 244 (89)	916 ± 212 (91)	-0.3 (-67, 67)	-15 (-82, 53)
	4 mo	1374 ± 276 (86)	1335 ± 273 (87)	39 (-43, 121)	44 (-39, 128)
	12 mo	1923 ± 437 (85)	1863 ± 422 (80)	60 (-71, 191)	54 (-78, 185)
Fat mass [%]	3-5 d	14.0 ± 2.7 (84)	13.7 ± 2.7 (84)	0.3 (-0.5, 1.1)	0.4 (-0.5, 1.2)
	6 wk	18.8 ± 3.3 (89)	19.2 ± 2.7 (91)	-0.4 (-1.2, 0.5)	-0.4 (-1.3, 0.5)
	4 mo	21.1 ± 2.8 (87)	21.1 ± 2.8 (87)	0.0 (-0.8, 0.9)	0.2 (-0.6, 1.1)
	12 mo	19.7 ± 3.0 (85)	19.7 ± 2.8 (80)	-0.0 (-0.9, 0.9)	0.0 (-0.9, 0.9)
Subscapular /Triceps	3-5 d	0.95 ± 0.16 (84)	0.98 ± 0.18 (84)	-0.03 (0.02, -0.08)	
	6 wk	0.93 ± 0.15 (89)	0.96 ± 0.19 (91)	-0.03 (0.02, -0.08)	
	4 mo	0.83 ± 0.15 (87)	0.87 ± 0.21 (87)	-0.04 (0.01, -0.10)	
	12 mo	0.80 ± 0.15 (86)	0.84 ± 0.18 (83)	-0.04 (0.01, -0.09)	
Trunk-to-total SFT	3-5 d	48.5 ± 3.2 (84)	48.8 ± 3.4 (84)	-0.3 (0.7, -1.3)	
	6 wk	49.6 ± 3.4 (89)	50.1 ± 3.6 (91)	-0.6 (0.5, -1.6)	
	4 mo	48.7 ± 3.7 (87)	49.4 ± 4.4 (87)	-0.7 (0.5, -1.9)	
	12 mo	45.0 ± 3.8 (85)	45.5 ± 4.0 (80)	-0.5 (0.7, -1.7)	

[1] Data are presented as mean ± SD (n) along with the non-adjusted mean difference (95% confidence interval). The last column gives the adjusted mean difference (95% CI) from multiple regression analysis (F-test, ANCOVA) controlling for sex and pregnancy duration in the analysis at birth, 6 weeks and 4 months and additionally for Ponderal Index at birth and breastfeeding status at 4 months in the analysis of the 1 year olds. There were no significant differences between groups in non-adjusted mean difference (Student´s t-test, p< 0.05) or adjusted mean difference (F-test, ANCOVA, p< 0.05).

Results

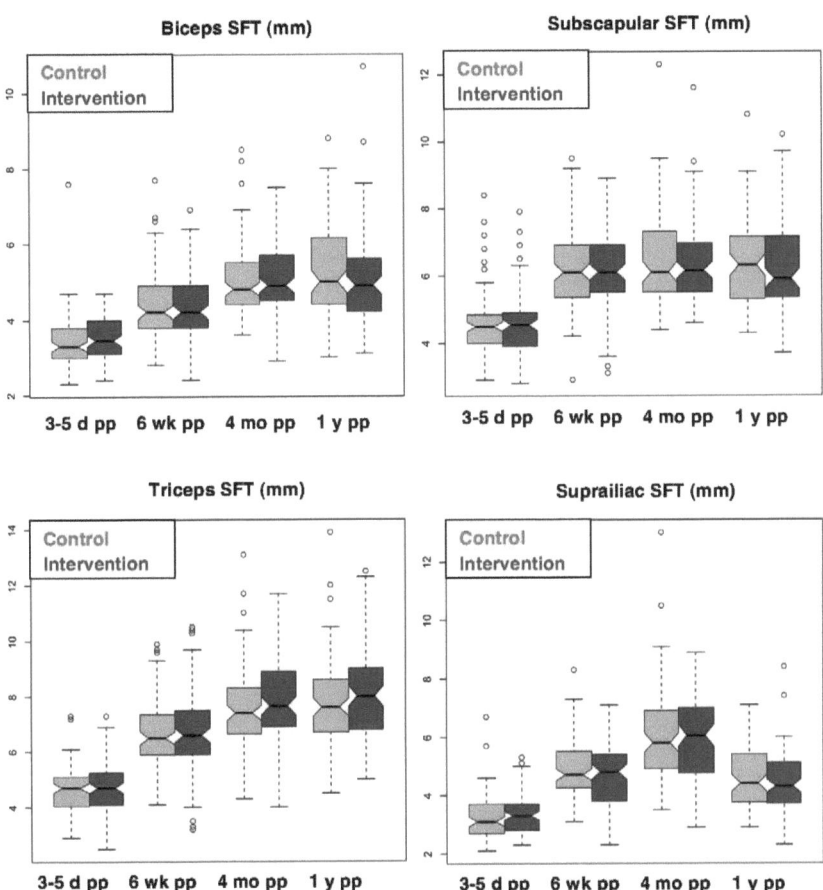

Figure 19: Individual SFT during the first year of life.
Data are presented as notched box-plots. Notched box-plots apply a "notch" or narrowing of the box around the median. Bottom and top edges of the box are located at 25th and 75th percentiles, center horizontal line is drawn at the median, whiskers mark the maximum and minimum. Outliners are shown as dots. There were no significant differences between groups (Mann-Whitney-U test p> 0.05)

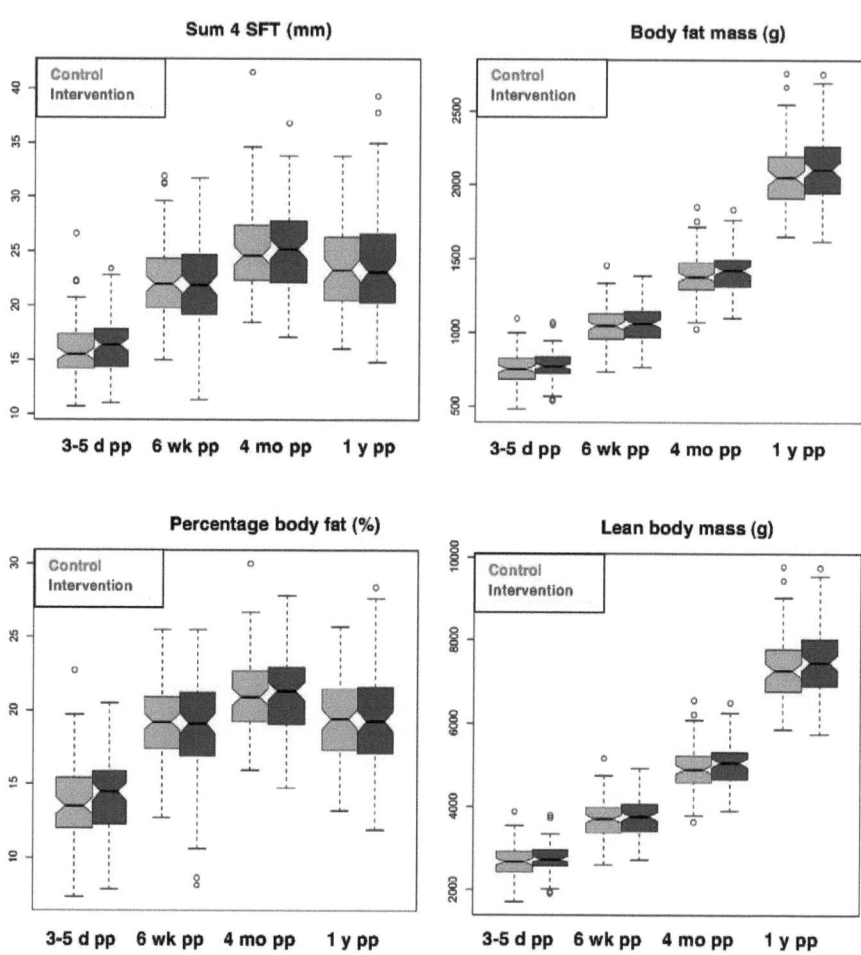

Figure 20: Infant body composition assessed by SFT during the first year of life. Data are presented as notched box-plots. Notched box-plots apply a "notch" or narrowing of the box around the median. Bottom and top edges of the box are located at 25th and 75th percentiles, center horizontal line is drawn at the median, whiskers mark the maximum and minimum. Outliners are shown as dots. There were no significant differences between groups (Mann-Whitney-U test p> 0.05)

Table 6: Adipose tissue growth and abdominal fat distribution during the first year of life assessed by ultrasonography[1]

		Intervention group mean ± SD (n)	Control group mean ± SD (n)	Unadjusted mean difference (95 % CI)	Adjusted mean difference (95% CI)
Age [days] at ultrsound	6 wk	45.4 ± 7.6 (80)	45.1 ± 7.4 (82)	-0.3 (-2.6, 2.0)	
	4 mo	110.9 ± 7.4 (79)	111.5 ± 9.6 (80)	0.5 (-2.1, 3.2)	
	12 mo	379.8 ± 18.6 (80)	380.2 ± 18.3 (78)	0.40 (-5.4, 6.2)	
Subcutaneous-area sagittal [mm²]	6 wk	30.5 ± 13.8 (77)	31.1 ± 10.9 (81)	-0.6 (-4.5, 3.3)	-0.4 (-3.6, 2.8)
	4 mo	41.9 ± 15.6 (77)	41.2 ± 14.7 (78)	0.7 (4.1, 5.5)	-1.0 (-5.2, 3.1)
	12 mo	28.6 ± 13.8 (77)	28.2 ± 12.8 (77)	0.5 (-3.8, 4.7)	-1.2 (-4.7, 2.3)
Subcutaneous-area axial [mm²]	6 wk	30.4 ± 13.5 (78)	30.7 ± 11.6 (82)	-0.3 (-4.2, 3.6)	-0.3 (-3.4, 2.9)
	4 mo	44.8 ± 16.0 (79)	44.9 ± 17.3 (79)	-0.1 (-5.3, 5.1)	-1.9 (-6.4, 2.6)
	12 mo	30.7 ± 14.2 (79)	32.3 ± 16.6 (77)	-1.6 (-6.4, 3.2)	-2.6 (-6.8, 1.7)
Preperitoneal-area sagittal [mm²]	6 wk	10.6 ± 4.2 (76)	10.8 ± 3.2 (76)	-0.2 (-1.4, 1.0)	-0.2 (-1.4, 1.0)
	4 mo	12.9 ± 3.6 (74)	13.2 ± 4.4 (74)	-0.2 (-1.6, 1.1)	-0.4 (-1.7, 0.9)
	12 mo	17.6 ± 5.3 (76)	18.2 ± 6.2 (77)	-0.6 (-2.4, 1.3)	-1.1 (-2.8, 0.7)
Ratio SC/PP	6 wk	3.04 ± 1.52 (76)	3.05 ± 1.16 (76)	-0.01 (-0.45, 0.42)	-0.00 (-0.38, 0.38)
	4 mo	3.60 ± 1.44 (74)	3.59 ± 1.52 (74)	0.01 (-0.47, 0.49)	-0.07 (-0.54, 0.41)
	12 mo	1.71 ± 0.68 (76)	1.76 ± 0.83 (77)	-0.06 (-0.30, 0.19)	-0.12 (-0.34, 0.10)

[1] Data are presented as mean ± SD (n) along with the non-adjusted mean difference (95% confidence interval). The last column gives the adjusted mean difference (95% CI) from multiple regression analysis (F-test, ANCOVA) controlling current weight and height at investigation. There were no significant differences between groups in non-adjusted mean difference (Student's t-test, $p < 0.05$) or adjusted mean difference (F-test, ANCOVA, $p < 0.05$).

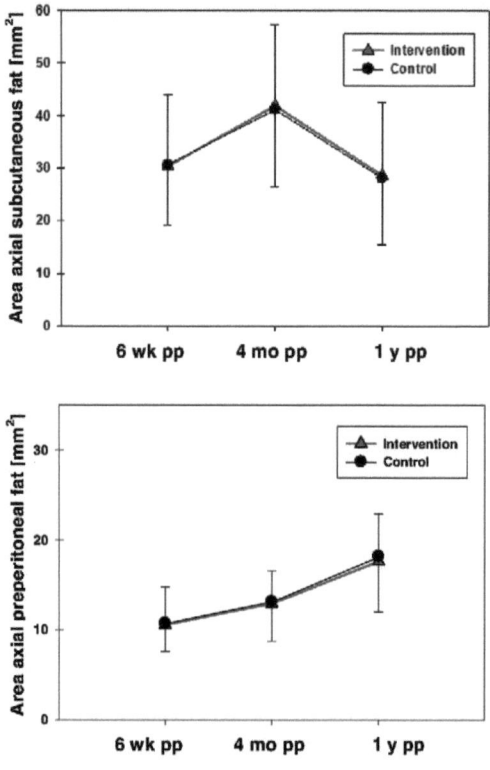

Figure 21: Development of abdominal subcutaneous and preperitoneal fat mass over the first year of life. Data are presented as mean ± SD. Intervention group=triangle; magenta.Control group=dot; black.

4.1.7 Subgroup analysis

<u>Sex</u>

Explanatory analysis (unpowered) showed no evidence of an interaction of the group effect and sex in the multivariable analysis for growth and fat mass (data not shown); thus, separate considerations of sex effects within groups were not indicated.

Breastfeeding

The post hoc subgroup analysis did not reveal consistently relevant [different signs (+ or -) of effect estimates over the course of follow-up] or statistically significant results regarding group differences in exclusively breastfed, partially breastfed, and exclusively formula-fed infants (data not shown).

4.2 Maternal and cord blood fatty acid profile in relation to infant body composition

The results on maternal and cord blood fatty acid profile and its relationship to infant body composition were described in Paper II.

4.2.1 Sample collection

Maternal blood plasma PLs and RBCs samples were available from 205 women at study entry (out of n=208 women randomized), 187/188 (PLs/RBCs) at 32nd wk of gestation (out of n=189 women in the study at 32nd wk of gestation), 148/148 (PLs/RBCs) at 6th wk pp (out of n= 162 women breastfeeding at 6th week pp) and 125/122 (PLs/RBCs) at 4 months pp (out of 141 women still breastfeeding at 4 months pp).

4.2.2 Maternal fatty acid profile over the course of pregnancy and lactation

Table 7 shows the phospholipid fatty acid composition of RBCs at 15th and 32nd week of gestation and at 6 weeks and 4 months pp as percentage of total fatty acids (% of total FAs). At study entry, there were no statistically significant differences in the fatty acid composition of RBCs and plasma PLs between the intervention and the control group (**Appendix 2 and 3**). Supplementation with fish oil and the concomitant AA-balanced diet starting from the 15th week of gestation onwards until 4 months pp resulted in a significant increase in the percentage of EPA,

DHA, and the sum of n-3 LCPUFAs in maternal RBCs at 32nd week of pregnancy and at 6 weeks and 4 months pp compared to the control group (Table 7, Appendix 2). In contrast, the proportions of AA and n-6 LCPUFAs in RBCs were significantly lower in the intervention group at 32nd week of pregnancy and throughout lactation compared to the control group (Table 7, Appendix 2).

Thus, the intervention resulted in a remarkable, significant decrease of the AA/DHA and the n-6/n-3 LCPUFs ratio in maternal RBCs at 32nd week of gestation, 6 weeks and 4 months pp compared with control subjects. Similar changes were obtained by analyzing the fatty acid profile of maternal plasma PLs (Appendix 3).

LCPUFAs levels in maternal RBCs correlated strongly and significantly with their respective LCPUFAs content in maternal plasma PLs at the 15th and 32nd week of gestation as well as at 6th week and 4th month pp (data not shown). In particular, the maternal erythrocyte n-6/n-3 LCPUFAs ratio was highly correlated with the plasma PLs n-6/n-3 LCPUFAs ratio at the 15th (r=0.717; n=204), the 32nd (r= 0.799; n=186) week of gestation, the 6th week (r=0.807; n=148) and 4th (r=0.865; n=123) month pp (all p<0.001).

4.2.3 Cord blood fatty acid profile

Table 8 illustrates the fatty acid composition of umbilical cord blood RBCs and plasma PLs as percentage of total fatty acids (% of total FAs). Umbilical cord RBCs samples were available from 132 newborns (CG/IG= 65/67). The fatty acid profile in umbilical cord plasma PLs samples was analyzed in a subsample of 56 newborns (28/28), only, due to limited sample volume for fatty acid analyses.

In umbilical RBCs the EPA, DHA, and n-3 LCPUFAs contents were significantly higher in the intervention group than in the control group. Conversely, the AA/DHA ratio and the n-6/n-3s LCPUFAs ratio (**Appendix 4**) as well as MUFA contents were significantly lower in the intervention group compared to the control group. Umbilical RBCs contents of AA were comparable between groups (Table 8).

Taken together, n-3 LCPUFAs supplementation and the concomitant AA balanced diet resulted on average in 2.9 fold higher EPA levels, 1.6 fold higher DHA contents, similar AA levels and in a 0.6 fold lower n-6/n-3 LCPUFAs ratio in umbilical cord blood RBCs. Basically, the same picture was observed in the fatty acid profiles of plasma PLs (Table 8, Appendix 4), except for AA content, which was significantly reduced in umbilical plasma PLs in the intervention group.

In umbilical cord blood, the n-6/n-3 LCPUFAs ratio in plasma PLs was closely associated with the n-6/n-3 LCPUFAs ratio in RBCs ($r=0.608$; $n=56$; $p< 0.001$).

We also explored the impact of gender on the fatty acid profile. In a model with the respective fatty acid as dependent variable and group*sex interactions of the newborn as influencing factor, no significant interaction between sex and intervention was observed for the fatty acid values in umbilical cord blood at birth (**Table 9**).

Table 7: Maternal RBCs fatty acid profile

fatty acid	group	n	15th wk gest mean ± SD	n	32nd wk gest mean ± SD	n	6th wk pp mean ± SD	n	16th wk pp mean ± SD
18:2n-6, LA	C	102	7.62 ± 0.98	95	6.91 ± 1.60	73	8.08 ± 1.48	58	8.45 ± 1.76
	I	103	7.39 ± 1.29	93	6.67 ± 1.34	75	7.84 ± 1.28	64	8.29 ± 1.37
18:3n-3, ALA	C	102	0.12 ± 0.03	95	0.13 ± 0.03	73	0.11 ± 0.02	59	0.10 ± 0.03
	I	103	0.12 ± 0.03	93	0.13 ± 0.04	75	0.10 ± 0.03	64	0.11 ± 0.03
20:3n-6, DHγLA	C	102	1.58 ± 0.35	95	1.47 ± 0.53	73	1.41 ± 0.44	59	1.41 ± 0.49
	I	102	1.56 ± 0.43	93	1.31 ± 0.41*	75	1.21 ± 0.42*	64	1.18 ± 0.37**
20:4n-6, AA†	C	102	12.51 ± 2.30	95	10.15 ± 3.89	73	11.37 ± 3.28	58	11.70 ± 3.90
	I	103	11.85 ± 3.09	93	8.82 ± 2.84***	75	9.43 ± 2.96***	64	9.98 ± 2.81***
20:5n-3, EPA†	C	102	0.41 ± 0.15	92	0.33 ± 0.16	72	0.50 ± 0.24	59	0.55 ± 0.28
	I	101	0.42 ± 0.18	93	0.66 ± 0.32***	74	0.83 ± 0.35***	64	0.94 ± 0.39***
22:4n-6, ADA	C	102	2.94 ± 0.67	95	2.43 ± 1.02	73	2.42 ± 0.79	59	2.39 ± 0.89
	I	103	2.73 ± 0.83	93	1.58 ± 0.59***	75	1.49 ± 0.56***	64	1.46 ± 0.51***
22:5n-3, DPA	C	102	2.02 ± 0.58	95	1.69 ± 0.91	73	1.79 ± 0.66	59	2.00 ± 0.93
	I	103	1.94 ± 0.69	93	1.54 ± 0.67	75	1.41 ± 0.56***	64	1.57 ± 0.57***
22:6n-3, DHA†	C	102	4.54 ± 1.24	95	4.34 ± 2.07	73	4.09 ± 1.52	59	3.29 ± 1.41
	I	103	4.56 ± 1.61	93	7.18 ± 2.97***	75	7.05 ± 2.70***	64	6.71 ± 2.37***
AA/DHA†	C	102	2.94 ± 0.75	95	2.79 ± 1.15	73	3.12 ± 1.01	59	4.05 ± 1.35
	I	103	2.95 ± 1.11	93	1.44 ± 0.63***	75	1.50 ± 0.48***	64	1.62 ± 0.43***
SAFA	C	102	47.14 ± 4.15	95	49.80 ± 8.45	73	48.36 ± 6.62	59	48.77 ± 7.46
	I	103	48.19 ± 6.42	93	49.91 ± 7.10	75	49.44 ± 6.85	64	49.14 ± 6.15*
MUFA	C	102	19.58 ± 1.35	95	21.27 ± 1.92	73	20.40 ± 1.41	59	19.83 ± 2.34
	I	103	19.78 ± 1.29	93	20.92 ± 1.70	75	19.98 ± 1.68	64	19.39 ± 1.71
PUFA	C	102	32.86 ± 5.10	95	28.52 ± 9.80	73	30.82 ± 7.74	59	30.94 ± 8.82
	I	102	31.55 ± 7.45	91	28.62 ± 8.43	75	30.15 ± 8.25	64	31.04 ± 7.61
n-3 LCPUFAs	C	102	7.05 ± 1.81	95	6.42 ± 3.05	73	6.44 ± 2.32	59	5.91 ± 2.44
	I	103	6.98 ± 2.36	93	9.46 ± 3.84***	75	9.33 ± 3.53***	64	9.27 ± 3.19***
n-6 LCPUFAs	C	102	18.02 ± 3.20	95	15.01 ± 5.64	73	16.11 ± 4.52	59	16.35 ± 5.32
	I	102	17.03 ± 4.37	91	12.40 ± 3.88***	75	12.82 ± 3.93***	64	13.31 ± 3.60***
n-6/n-3 LCPUFAs†	C	102	2.70 ± 0.64	95	2.80 ± 1.17	73	2.78 ± 0.89	59	3.14 ± 1.06
	I	102	2.76 ± 1.03	91	1.54 ± 0.63***	75	1.54 ± 0.53***	64	1.56 ± 0.43***

Data are presented as mean ± SD (n). Values for fatty acids are expressed as a percentage of the weight of the total fatty acids (% FA). Differences in fatty acid values between the groups were compared using the Mann-Whitney-U-Test ($p<0.05$). Changes in maternal fatty acid profile over time were determined by using the Friedman-Test ($p< 0.05$). All fatty acids showed significant change over time ($p<0.001$), except SAFA ($p=0.082$). Values marked with stars show significant differences between groups at the same time point (Mann-Whitney-U-Test, * $p< 0.05$; **$p<0.01$, ***$p<0.001$) after Bonferroni-corrections.† illustrated in Appendix 2.

SAFA: C4:0 – C27:0
MUFA: sum of all cis-FA with one double bound
PUFA: sum of all cis-FA with two or more double bounds
n-6 LCPUFAs: C20:2n-6; 20:3n-6; 20:4n-6; C22:2n-6; C22:4n-6; C22:5n-6
n-3 LCPUFAs: C20:3n-3; C20:4n-3; 20:5n-3; C21:5n-3; C22:3n-3; 22:5n-3; 22:6n-3

Table 8: Cord blood plasma PLs and RBCs fatty acid profile

fatty acid	group	n	Cord blood plasma PLs mean ± SD	n	Cord blood RBCs mean ± SD
18:2n-6, LA	C	28	6.36 ± 1.08	65	2.49 ± 1.30
	I	28	6.60 ± 0.82	67	2.68 ± 0.88*
18:3n-3, ALA	C	12	0.03 ± 0.01	62	0.06 ± 0.03
	I	19	0.04 ± 0.01	65	0.05 ± 0.03
20:3n-6, DHγLA	C	28	4.73 ± 0.88	65	1.46 ± 0.72
	I	28	4.66 ± 0.46	67	1.75 ± 0.90
20:4n-6, AA	C	28	17.93 ± 1.91	65	7.62 ± 4.85
	I	28	14.96 ± 1.64***	67	7.82 ± 4.35
20:5n-3, EPA	C	28	0.27 ± 0.12	56	0.08 ± 0.06
	I	28	0.93 ± 0.42***	65	0.23 ± 0.18***
22:4n-6 ADA	C	28	0.86 ± 0.19	65	1.75 ± 1.18
	I	28	0.68 ± 0.16**	67	1.76 ± 1.06
22:5n-3, DPA	C	28	0.42 ± 0.15	63	0.43 ± 0.70
	I	28	0.55 ± 0.18*	66	0.47 ± 0.31
22:6n-3, DHA	C	28	6.14 ± 1.54	65	2.54 ± 2.19
	I	28	8.28 ± 1.33***	67	3.95 ± 2.71**
AA/DHA†	C	28	3.11 ± 0.87	65	3.81 ± 1.11
	I	28	1.86 ± 0.41***	67	2.37 ± 0.77***
SAFA	C	28	47.81 ± 0.79	65	63.29 ± 9.08
	I	28	48.05 ± 0.80	67	61.43 ± 9.46
MUFA	C	28	13.41 ± 1.37	65	18.79 ± 1.64
	I	28	13.63 ± 1.52	67	18.28 ± 1.67*
PUFA	C	28	38.49 ± 1.42	65	17.49 ± 10.32
	I	28	37.99 ± 1.54	67	19.88 ± 10.53
n-3 LCPUFAs	C	28	6.88 ± 1.69	65	3.03 ± 2.62
	I	28	9.89 ± 1.51***	67	4.65 ± 3.17**
n-6 LCPUFAs	C	28	25.16 ± 1.47	65	12.03 ± 7.32
	I	28	21.41 ± 1.59***	67	12.46 ± 6.73
n-6/n-3 LCPUFAs†	C	28	3.92 ± 1.23	65	5.06 ± 1.74
	I	28	2.23 ± 0.45***	67	3.27 ± 1.34***

Data are presented as mean ± SD (n). Values for fatty acids are expressed as a percentage of the weight of the total fatty acids (%FA). Differences in fatty acid values between the groups were compared using the Mann-Whitney-U-Test ($p<0.05$). Values marked with stars show significant differences between groups (Mann-Whitney-U-Test, * $p< 0.05$; ** $p<0.01$, *** $p<0.001$). † illustrated in Appendix 4.

SAFA: C4:0 – C27:0
MUFA: sum of all cis-FA with one double bound
PUFA: sum of all cis-FA with two or more double bounds
n-6 LCPUFAs: C20:2n-6; 20:3n-6; 20:4n-6; C22:2n-6; C22:4n-6; C22:5n-6
n-3 LCPUFAs: C20:3n-3; C20:4n-3; 20:5n-3; C21:5n-3; C22:3n-3; 22:5n-3; 22:6n-3

Table 9: Cord blood RBCs fatty acid profile according to gender

fatty acid	group	n	Cord Blood all mean ± SD	n	male mean ± SD	n	female mean ± SD	g x
18:2n-6, LA	C	65	2.49 ± 1.30	30	2.28 ± 0.63	35	2.67 ± 1.66	0.987
	I	67	2.68 ± 0.88*	29	2.45 ± 0.77	38	2.85 ± 0.92	
18:3n-3, ALA	C	62	0.06 ± 0.03	30	0.07 ± 0.03	32	0.06 ± 0.03	0.953
	I	65	0.05 ± 0.03	29	0.05 ± 0.03	36	0.05 ± 0.03	
20:3n-6, DHγLA	C	65	1.46 ± 0.72	31	1.40 ± 0.68	34	1.51 ± 0.76	0.396
	I	67	1.75 ± 0.90	29	1.55 ± 0.88	38	1.91 ± 0.89	
20:4n-6, AA	C	65	7.62 ± 4.85	31	7.18 ± 4.65	34	8.02 ± 5.07	0.793
	I	67	7.82 ± 4.35	29	7.11 ± 4.61	38	8.37 ± 4.11	
20:5n-3, EPA	C	56	0.08 ± 0.06	26	0.07 ± 0.05	30	0.08 ± 0.07	0.542
	I	65	0.23 ± 0.18***	28	0.20 ± 0.18	37	0.25 ± 0.17	
22:4n-6, ADA	C	65	1.75 ± 1.18	31	1.57 ± 1.07	34	1.91 ± 1.26	0.894
	I	67	1.76 ± 1.06	29	1.60 ± 1.17	38	1.88 ± 0.96	
22:5n-3, DPA	C	63	0.43 ± 0.70	29	0.29 ± 0.19	34	0.55 ± 0.93	0.310
	I	66	0.47 ± 0.31	29	0.43 ± 0.34	37	0.49 ± 0.29	
22:6n-3, DHA	C	65	2.54 ± 2.19	31	2.26 ± 1.90	34	2.79 ± 2.43	0.224
	I	67	3.95 ± 2.71**	29	3.37 ± 2.71	38	4.39 ± 2.65	
AA/DHA	C	65	3.81 ± 1.11	31	3.87 ± 1.07	34	3.73 ± 1.17	0.427
	I	67	2.37 ± 0.77***	29	2.59 ± 0.89†	38	2.20 ± 0.62	
SAFA	C	65	63.29 ± 9.08	31	64.46 ± 8.39	34	62.22 ± 9.67	0.680
	I	67	61.43 ± 9.46	29	63.46 ±	38	59.88 ± 8.72	
MUFA	C	65	18.79 ± 1.64	31	18.92 ± 1.52	34	18.67 ± 1.76	0.717
	I	67	18.28 ± 1.67*	29	18.30 ± 1.36	38	18.26 ± 1.89	
PUFA	C	65	17.49 ± 10.32	31	16.14 ± 9.53	34	18.71 ±	0.782
	I	67	19.88 ± 10.53	29	17.85 ±	38	21.43 ±	
n-3 LCPUFAs	C	65	3.03 ± 2.62	31	2.60 ± 2.10	34	3.43 ± 3.00	0.761
	I	67	4.65 ± 3.17**	29	4.01 ± 3.21	38	5.14 ± 3.09	
n-6 LCPUFAs	C	65	12.03 ± 7.32	31	11.22 ± 6.89	34	12.76 ± 7.73	0.837
	I	67	12.46 ± 6.73	29	11.30 ± 7.17	38	13.34 ± 6.33	
n-6/n-3	C	65	5.06 ± 1.74	31	5.36 ± 1.80	34	4.78 ± 1.66	0.837
	I	67	3.27 ± 1.34***	29	3.53 ± 1.54	38	3.07 ± 1.15	

Data are presented as mean ± SD (n). Values for fatty acids are expressed as a percentage of the weight of the total fatty acids (% FA). Differences in fatty acid values between the groups were compared using the Mann-Whitney-U-Test (p<0.05). Values marked with stars show significant differences between groups (Mann-Whitney-U-Test, * p< 0.05; **p<0.01, ***p<0.001). Values marked with a cross show significantly different distribution between boys and girls in the within group comparison (Mann-Whitney-U-Test). There were no significant interactions between sex and group.

SAFA: C4:0 – C27:0
MUFA: sum of all cis-FA with one double bound
PUFA: sum of all cis-FA with two or more double bounds
n-6 LCPUFAs: C20:2n-6; 20:3n-6; 20:4n-6; C22:2n-6; C22:4n-6; C22:5n-6
n-3 LCPUFAs: C20:3n-3; C20:4n-3; 20:5n-3; C21:5n-3; C22:3n-3; 22:5n-3; 22:6n-3

4.2.4 Relationship between maternal fatty acid profile at 32nd week of gestation and cord blood fatty acid profile

The neonatal plasma PLs fatty acid levels (% of total FAs) of DHγLA, AA, ADA, DHA, the sum of n-6 and n-3 LCPUFAs, and the sum of SAFA, as well as the AA/DHA ratio and the n-6/n-3 LCPUFAs ratio were higher than the levels in maternal plasma, while in most of the cases, the neonatal RBCs FA proportions were lower than the maternal RBCs FA proportions throughout pregnancy.

Maternal plasma PLs AA, DHA, EPA, AA/DHA ratio, total n-3 LCPUFAs, total n-6 LCPUFAs and the n-6/n-3 LCPUFAs ratio at 32nd week of gestation were significantly positively correlated with the respective fatty acid levels and ratios in umbilical cord blood PLs (e.g. n-6/n-3 LCPUFAs ratio: r=0.804, p< 0.01). Most correlations between maternal and cord blood fatty acids in RBCs were significant, except for AA and n-6 LCPUFAs, but clearly less pronounced than in the PLs (**Table 10**).

Table 10: Correlation coefficients between A) maternal RBCs fatty acid profile at 32nd week of gestation and cord blood RBCs fatty acid profile and B) maternal plasma PLs fatty acid profile at 32nd week of gestation and cord blood plasma PLs

A)

Maternal RBCs 32nd wk gest ~ cord blood RBCs		
fatty acid	n	r
AA	132	0.104
DHA	132	0.265**
EPA	121	0.412***
AA/DHA	132	0.657***
n-3 LCPUFAs	132	0.266**
n-6 LCPUFAs	132	0.100
n-6/n-3 LCPUFAs	132	0.672 **

B)

Maternal plasma PLs 32nd wk gest ~ cord blood plasma PLs		
fatty acid	n	r
AA	56	0.726 **
DHA	56	0.634 **
EPA	56	0.739 **
AA/DHA	56	0.755 **
n-3 LCPUFAs	56	0.744***
n-6 LCPUFAs	56	0.738***
n-6/n-3 LCPUFAs	56	0.804 **

Data are presented as Spearman correlation coefficients. Values marked with stars show significant correlations between the respective fatty acid in maternal and umbilical cord blood (Spearman: **p<0.01, ***p<0.001).

4.2.5 Relationship between maternal LCPUFAs profile and pregnancy duration

Maternal plasma PLs DHA and EPA concentration and the sum of n-3 LCPUFAs at 32nd week of gestation were significantly correlated with pregnancy duration (DHA: n= 187, r=0.184, p=0.012; EPA: n=187, r=0.270, p < 0.001; n-3 LCPUFAs: n=187, r=0.209, p=0.004). Maternal RBCs AA and total n-6 LCPUFAs were significantly negatively correlated with pregnancy duration (AA: n=187, r= -0.144, p<0.05; n-6 LCPUFAs: r= -0.141, p<0.05) in the unadjusted analysis.

4.2.6 Maternal LCPUFAs profile in relation to infant growth parameters and fat mass

Potential influences of the maternal RBCs fatty acid profile at 32nd week of gestation on infant growth up to 1 year pp or infant body composition assessed by SFT measurements and abdominal sonography were explored by means of multiple regression models and partial correlations. Results were controlled for gestational age, parity, infant sex and group in the analysis at birth, and additionally for Ponderal Index at birth and breastfeeding status in the analysis of the 6 weeks, 4 months or 1 year olds. The fatty acid profile in these analyses comprised DHA, EPA, n-3 LCPUFAs, AA, n-6 LCPUFAs content in RBCs as well as RBCs AA/DHA and n-6/n-3 LCPUFAs ratio. Data are shown for DHA, n-3 LCPUFAs, AA, and n-6 LCPUFAs, only.

Maternal RBCs DHA, total n-3 LCPUFAs and total n-6 LCPUFAs at the 32nd week of gestation were significantly positively related with birth weight (p<0.05) in analyses corrected for relevant confounders, such as pregnancy duration, parity, sex, and group (**Table 11**). For instance, 1 unit increment of RBCs DHA at 32nd week of pregnancy (% of total FA) resulted in a 24.4 g (adjusted beta) higher birth weight in the adjusted analyses (p< 0.05). Total RBCs n-3 LCPUFAs, AA and total n-6 LCPUFAs were significantly positively associated with length at birth and except for AA also with head circumference at birth (p<0.05, Table 11).

The n-6/n-3 LCPUFAs ratio at 32nd week of gestation was significantly negatively related to length at birth (-0.36 [95%: CI -0.69, -0.03]; p=0.034).

Maternal RBCs EPA (data not shown), DHA, n-3 LCPUFAs, AA and n-6 LCPUFAs at 32nd week of gestation were significantly positively related with newborn lean body mass (g) at birth when corrected for gestational age, parity, sex and group (**Table 12**). Maternal RBCs n-3 LCPUFAs were significantly positively related to fat mass (g) at birth in the adjusted analysis.

Maternal RBCs AA and total n-6 LCPUFAs were significantly negatively related to BMI (Table 11) and Ponderal Index at 1 y pp (e.g. RBCs AA 32nd wk ~ Ponderal Index 1y: ßadj -0.11 [95%: CI -0.19, -0.02]; r= -0.16; p=0.016; RBCs n-6 LCPUFAs 32nd wk ~ Ponderal Index 1y: ßadj -0.08 [95%: CI -0.14, -0.02]; r= -0.17; p=0.008).

Importantly, neither the maternal RBCs DHA, EPA, AA, n-3 LCPUFAs, n-6 LCPUFAs nor the AA/DHA or the n-6/n-3 LCPUFAs ratio were consistently associated with individual skinfold thicknesses (data not shown), the sum of the four skinfolds (Table 12), or measures of abdominal ultrasonography (**Table 13**) at any time point studied during the first year of life (e.g. n-6/n-3 LCPUFAs ratio RBCs 32nd week ~ sum 4 SFT 1 y: ßadj -0.17 [-0.69, 0.34]; r=-0.03; p=0.516).

Table 11: Final adjusted multiple regression analysis and partial correlation coefficients on the effect of maternal RBCs fatty acid profile (at 32nd week of gestation) on infant growth and growth indices[1]

	n	RBCs DHA 32nd wk adj beta (95% CI)	r	RBCs n-3 LCPUFA 32nd wk adj beta (95% CI)	r	RBCs AA 32nd wk adj beta (95% CI)	r	n	RBCs n-6 LCPUFAs 32nd wk adj beta (95% CI)	r
Weight at birth [g]	187	24.38 (0.42, 48.33)	0.22*	20.38 (2.78, 37.99)	0.24*	17.25 (-0.58, 35.09)	0.11	185	12.51 (-0.12, 25.14)	0.10*
6th week	177	24.16 (-8.96, 57.29)	0.13	21.53 (-2.81, 45.86)	0.16	17.79 (-6.74, 42.32)	0.09	175	12.20 (-5.08, 29.47)	0.09
4 months	172	19.72 (-19.25, 58.69)	0.13	15.17 (-13.49, 43.84)	0.13	6.82 (-22.33, 35.97)	0.00	170	4.43 (-16.23, 25.1)	0.02
12 months	169	-0.99 (-58.1, 56.12)	-0.05	1.40 (-40.7, 43.5)	0.05	-26.56 (-68.99, 15.88)	-0.13	167	-16.45 (-46.53, 13.64)	-0.13
Length at birth [cm]	187	0.12 (-0.01, 0.24)	0.15	0.10 (0.01, 0.19)	0.17*	0.10 (0.01, 0.19)	0.13*	185	0.07 (0.00, 0.13)	0.12*
6th week	177	0.05 (-0.07, 0.18)	0.10	0.05 (-0.04, 0.15)	0.11	0.07 (-0.03, 0.16)	0.07	175	0.05 (-0.02, 0.12)	0.07
4 months	173	0.03 (-0.09, 0.15)	0.05	0.02 (-0.07, 0.11)	0.05	0.03 (-0.05, 0.12)	0.02	171	0.03 (-0.03, 0.09)	0.03
12 months	169	0.07 (-0.08, 0.22)	0.08	0.04 (-0.07, 0.15)	0.06	0.05 (-0.07, 0.16)	0.00	167	0.05 (-0.03, 0.12)	0.01
HC at birth [cm]	187	0.07 (0.00, 0.14)	0.15	0.06 (0.00, 0.12)	0.19*	0.05 (0.00, 0.11)	0.12	185	0.04 (0.00, 0.08)	0.13*
6th week	177	0.02 (-0.04, 0.1)	0.04	0.02 (-0.02, 0.07)	0.07	0.02 (-0.02, 0.07)	0.04	175	0.02 (-0.02, 0.05)	0.04
4 months	172	0.02 (-0.04, 0.09)	0.06	0.03 (-0.02, 0.08)	0.09	0.02 (-0.03, 0.07)	0.01	170	0.01 (-0.02, 0.05)	0.01
12 months	169	0.01 (-0.08, 0.1)	0.07	0.01 (-0.05, 0.08)	0.07	-0.02 (-0.09, 0.04)	-0.11	167	-0.01 (-0.06, 0.03)	-0.11
BMI at birth [kg/m²]	187	0.04 (-0.03, 0.1)	0.18	0.03 (-0.02, 0.08)	0.19	0.02 (-0.03, 0.07)	0.03	185	0.02 (-0.02, 0.05)	0.02
6th week	177	0.05 (-0.02, 0.12)	0.10	0.04 (-0.01, 0.09)	0.12	0.02 (-0.03, 0.08)	0.07	175	0.01 (-0.03, 0.05)	0.06
4 months	172	0.04 (-0.04, 0.12)	0.12	0.03 (-0.03, 0.09)	0.12	-0.00 (-0.06, 0.06)	0.02	170	-0.00 (-0.05, 0.04)	-0.05
12 months	169	-0.04 (-0.11, 0.04)	-0.01	-0.02 (-0.08, 0.04)	-0.01	-0.07 (-0.13, -0.01)	-0.18*	167	-0.05 (-0.09, -0.01)	-0.18*

[1] Data are presented as the regression coefficient of the fatty acid of interest (β) along with the (95% confidence interval)) and the partial correlation coefficient according to Spearman (r) of the fatty acid of interest. At the time point of birth results were corrected for pregnancy duration, group, parity and sex. At 6 weeks pp, 4 month pp and 1 year pp, correction was performed for following variables: pregnancy duration, group, parity, sex, Ponderal index at birth and breastfeeding status at the respective time point. Breastfeeding status at 4 months was used in the analysis of the 1 year olds as it reflects the last time point of assessment. The stars indicate significant total model p-values of the (final) multivariable-adjusted analysis (F-test, ANCOVA, p< 0.05) and in the Spearman correlation coefficient (p< 0.05).

Results

Table 12: Final adjusted multiple regression analysis and partial correlation coefficients on the effect of maternal RBCs fatty acid profile (at 32nd week of gestation) on infant adipose tissue growth assessed by skinfold thickness measurements[1]

	n	RBCs DHA 32nd wk		RBCs n-3 LCPUFAs 32nd wk		n	RBCs AA 32nd wk		RBCs n-6 LCPUFAs 32nd wk	
		adj beta (95% CI)	r	adj beta (95% CI)	r		adj beta (95% CI)	r	adj beta (95% CI)	r
Sum 4 SFT birth [mm]	168	0.11 (-0.04, 0.27)	0.14	0.08 (-0.03, 0.2)	0.14	166	0.06 (-0.06, 0.18)	0.08	0.05 (-0.03, 0.13)	0.09
6th week	177	0.06 (-0.17, 0.28)	0.04	0.05 (-0.11, 0.22)	0.06	175	0.08 (-0.11, 0.22)	0.08	0.05 (-0.07, 0.17)	0.09
4 months	172	0.02 (-0.22, 0.27)	0.03	0.03 (-0.15, 0.21)	0.04	170	0.03 (-0.15, 0.22)	0.05	0.03 (-0.1, 0.16)	0.06
12 months	164	0.11 (-0.15, 0.36)	0.08	0.08 (-0.11, 0.26)	0.09	162	-0.01 (-0.2, 0.19)	-0.03	-0.01 (-0.14, 0.13)	-0.03
Fat mass at birth [g]	168	7.97 (-0.25, 16.18)	0.19	6.19 (0.11, 12.26)	0.20*	166	4.85 (-1.35, 11.04)	0.11	3.75 (-0.62, 8.11)	0.12
6th week	177	6.26 (-7.02, 19.54)	0.08	5.75 (-4.02, 15.52)	0.10	175	5.20 (-4.63, 15.03)	0.09	3.83 (-3.09, 10.76)	0.09
4 months	171	4.27 (-12.1, 20.62)	0.08	3.67 (-8.36, 15.71)	0.09	169	2.24 (-9.96, 14.44)	0.02	1.79 (-6.88, 10.45)	0.02
12 months	164	7.80 (-17.62, 33.22)	0.25	6.38 (-12.43, 25.20)	0.10	162	-5.16 (-24.58, 14.26)	-0.04	-3.02 (-16.9, 10.86)	-0.03
Lean mass at birth [g]	168	21.85 (3.62, 40.07)	0.23*	18.00 (4.56, 31.43)	0.20**	166	14.72 (0.96, 28.46)	0.13*	10.66 (0.92, 20.39)	0.12*
6th week	177	17.90 (-4.73, 40.53)	0.14	15.78 (-0.84, 32.4)	0.17	175	12.59 (-4.18, 29.36)	0.08	8.36 (-3.47, 20.19)	0.07
4 months	171	14.10 (-13.05, 41.26)	0.13	10.46 (-9.53, 30.44)	0.13	169	4.03 (-16.26, 24.32)	0.02	2.28 (-12.05, 16.61)	0.04
12 months	164	-3.36 (-42.75, 36.03)	-0.06	0.67 (-28.5, 29.83)	0.07	162	-17.11 (-47.08, 12.84)	-0.15	-9.48 (-30.7, 11.73)	-0.15
Body fat at birth [%]	168	0.11 (-0.05, 0.27)	0.14	0.08 (-0.03, 0.2)	0.14	166	0.06 (-0.06, 0.18)	0.09	0.05 (-0.03, 0.14)	0.10
6th week	177	0.05 (-0.13, 0.23)	0.03	0.05 (-0.09, 0.18)	0.05	175	0.06 (-0.08, 0.19)	0.10	0.05 (-0.05, 0.14)	0.11
4 months	172	0.02 (-0.14, 0.18)	0.03	0.02 (-0.1, 0.14)	0.04	171	0.02 (-0.1, 0.15)	0.05	0.02 (-0.07, 0.11)	0.06
12 months	164	0.08 (-0.1, 0.25)	0.08	0.05 (-0.07, 0.18)	0.09	162	-0.00 (-0.13, 0.13)	-0.03	-0.00 (-0.1, 0.09)	-0.03

[1] Data are presented as the regression coefficient of the fatty acid of interest (β) along with the (95% confidence interval) and the partial correlation coefficient according to Spearman (r) of the fatty acid of interest. At the time point of birth results were corrected for pregnancy duration, group, parity and sex. At 6 weeks pp, 4 month pp and 1 year pp, correction was performed for following variables: pregnancy duration, group, parity, sex, Ponderal index at birth and breastfeeding status at the respective time point. Breastfeeding status at 4 months was used in the analysis of the 1 year olds as it reflects the last time point of assessment. The stars indicate significant total model p-values of the (final) multivariable-adjusted analysis (F-test, ANCOVA, p< 0.05) and in the Spearman correlation coefficient (p< 0.05).

Table 13: Final adjusted multiple regression analysis and partial correlation coefficients on the effect of maternal RBCs fatty acid status (at 32nd week of gestation) on infant adipose tissue growth assessed by ultrasonography[1]

	n	RBCs DHA 32nd wk adj beta (95% CI)	r	RBCs n-3 LCPUFAs 32nd wk adj beta (95% CI)	r	n	RBCs AA 32nd wk adj beta (95% CI)	r	RBCs n-6 LCPUFAs 32nd wk adj beta (95% CI)	r
A sag sc [mm²]										
6th week	156	-0.00 (-0.01, 0.01)	0.00	0.00 (-0.01, 0.00)	0.00	154	-0.00 (-0.01, 0.00)	-0.01	-0.00 (0.00, 0.00)	-0.03
4 months	153	-0.00 (-0.01, 0.01)	-0.04	-0.00 (-0.01, 0.01)	-0.03	151	-0.00 (-0.01, 0.01)	0.00	-0.00 (-0.01, 0.00)	-0.01
12 months	154	0.00 (-0.01, 0.01)	0.06	0.00 (0.00, 0.01)	0.07	152	-0.00 (-0.01, 0.01)	-0.01	-0.00 (0.00, 0.00)	-0.02
A ax sc [mm²]										
6th week	158	-0.00 (-0.01, 0.01)	-0.02	-0.00 (-0.01, 0.00)	-0.03	156	0.00 (-0.01, 0.01)	0.05	0.00 (0.00, 0.00)	0.06
4 months	156	-0.00 (-0.01, 0.01)	0.00	-0.00 (-0.01, 0.01)	0.00	154	-0.00 (-0.01, 0.01)	-0.01	-0.00 (-0.01, 0.01)	-0.03
12 months	156	0.00 (-0.01, 0.01)	0.00	0.00 (-0.01, 0.01)	0.01	154	-0.00 (-0.01, 0.01)	-0.02	-0.00 (-0.01, 0.00)	-0.03
A sag pp [mm²]										
6th week	150	0.00 (0.00, 0.00)	-0.02	0.00 (0.00, 0.00)	0.04	148	-0.00 (0.00, 0.00)	-0.02	0.00 (0.00, 0.00)	-0.01
4 months	146	-0.00 (0.00, 0.00)	-0.04	-0.00 (0.00, 0.00)	-0.04	144	-0.00 (0.00, 0.00)	-0.06	-0.00 (0.00, 0.00)	-0.07
12 months	153	-0.00 (0.00, 0.00)	-0.05	0.00 (0.00, 0.00)	-0.03	151	-0.00 (0.00, 0.00)	-0.04	-0.00 (0.00, 0.00)	-0.05
Ratio SC/PP										
6th week	148	-0.00 (-0.09, 0.09)	-0.02	-0.01 (-0.07, 0.06)	-0.01	146	0.01 (-0.05, 0.08)	0.06	0.02 (-0.03, 0.06)	0.08
4 months	146	0.03 (-0.06, 0.13)	0.07	0.03 (-0.05, 0.01)	0.07	144	0.04 (-0.03, 0.11)	0.10	0.03 (-0.02, 0.08)	0.11
12 months	151	0.01 (-0.04, 0.05)	0.03	0.00 (-0.03, 0.04)	0.03	149	-0.00 (-0.04, 0.03)	-0.03	0.00 (-0.03, 0.02)	-0.04

[1] Data are presented as the regression coefficient of the fatty acid of interest (β) along with the (95% confidence interval) and the partial correlation coefficient according to Spearman (r) of the fatty acid of interest. At the time point of birth results were corrected for pregnancy duration, group, parity and sex. At 6 weeks pp, 4 month pp and 1 year pp, correction was performed for following variables: pregnancy duration, group, parity, sex, Ponderal index at birth and breastfeeding status at the respective time point. Breastfeeding status at 4 months was used in the analysis of the 1 year olds as it reflects the last time point of assessment. The stars indicate significant total model p-values of the (final) multivariable-adjusted analysis (F-test, ANCOVA, p< 0.05) and in the Spearman correlation coefficient (p< 0.05).

4.2.7 Neonatal LCPUFAs in relation to infant growth parameters and fat mass

We also examined the relationship between the neonatal RBCs fatty acid profile and infant outcomes from birth up to 1 year of age.

Neonatal EPA and n-3 LCPUFAs were significantly negatively related with the subscapular skinfold thickness, percentage body fat and body fat mass (g) at birth, when corrected for pregnancy duration, parity, sex and group (**Table 14**). For instance, 1 unit increment of RBCs EPA in umbilical cord blood (% of total FA) resulted in a 2.1 mm (adjusted beta) lower subscapular SFT in the adjusted analyses (r=-0.28; p= 0.001, n=114). Cord blood EPA was significantly related with the sum of 4 SFT at birth (ßadj -4.49 [95% CI -7.96, -1.01]; r=-0.21; p=0.013, n=114), also. Neonatal DHA was significantly negatively related to percentage body fat, only (ßadj -0.20 [95%CI -0.40, 0.00]; r=-0.17; p=0.049, n=125). The n-6/n-3 LCPUFAs ratio in umbilical RBCs was significantly positively related to BMI at birth (ßadj 0.14 [95% CI 0.02, 0.27], r=0.04; p=0.030, n=113), though the relationship was weakly. Neonatal RBCs DHA, AA, n-3 LCPUFAs and n-6 LCPUFAs were significantly negatively related to Ponderal Index and BMI at 6 weeks pp (data not shown). However, this association was not significant at any later stages up to 1 y of life (data not shown). Neonatal RBCs AA and total n-6 LCPUFAs were significantly positively associated with the ratio between SC/PP adipose tissue assessed by abdominal ultrasonography at 4 months pp, but this effect was not detectable at 6 weeks pp or at 1 year pp (data not shown).Neither neonatal RBCs DHA, EPA, AA, n-3 LCPUFAs, n-6 LCPUFAs nor the n-6/n-3 LCPUFAs or AA/DHA ratio were significantly correlated with the individual skinfold thicknesses, the sum of the four skinfolds or parameters of fat mass at 1 y pp (**Appendix 5**).

Table 14: Final adjusted multiple regression model and partial correlation coefficients on the effect of cord blood RBCs fatty acid status on infant growth and body fat mass at birth[1]

		cord RBCs EPA			cord RBCs n-3 LCPUFAs	
	n	adj beta (95% CI)	r	n	adj beta (95% CI)	r
Birth weight [g]	121	-423.80 (-988.97, 141.38)	-0.03	132	-17.40 (-42.26, 7.40)	-0.03
Birth length [cm]	121	-1.96 (-4.77, 0.84)	-0.03	132	-0.07 (-0.2, 0.05)	0.00
HC at birth [cm]	121	0.01 (-1.7, 1.72)	0.08	132	-0.01 (-0.08, 0.06)	-0.07
BMI [kg/m²]	121	-0.62 (-2.15, 0.92)	-0.08	132	-0.03 (-0.1, 0.04)	-0.04
PI [kg/m³]	121	-0.28 (-3.52, 2.97)	-0.09	132	-0.02 (-0.17, 0.13)	-0.04
Biceps SFT [mm]	114	-0.66 (-1.58, 0.27)	-0.14	125	-0.03 (-0.07, 0.01)	-0.12
TricepsSFT [mm]	114	-0.79 (-1.97, 0.40)	-0.07	125	-0.02 (-0.08, 0.03)	-0.05
Subscapular SFT [mm]	114	-2.11 (-3.29, -0.93)	-0.28***	125	-0.06 (-0.12, 0.00)	-0.19*
Suprailiac SFT [mm]	114	-0.94 (-1.91, 0.04)	-0.18	125	-0.03 (-0.08, 0.01)	-0.15
Sum 4 SFT [mm]²	114	-4.49 (-7.96, -1.01)	-0.21*	125	-0.15 (-0.31, 0.02)	-0.16
Fat mass [g]³	114	-242.37 (-429.69, -55.05)	-0.15*	125	-8.73 (-17.25, -0.21)	-0.12*
Lean mass [g]³	114	-255.60 (-685.74, 174.54)	0.08	125	-13.72 (-32.64, 5.19)	-0.04
Fat mass [% bw]³	114	-5.05 (-8.61, -1.48)	-0.22**	125	-0.17 (-0.34, 0.00)	-0.17*

[1] Data are presented as the regression coefficient of the fatty acid of interest (β) along with the (95% confidence interval) and the partial correlation coefficient according to Spearman (r) of the fatty acid of interest. At the time point of birth results were corrected for pregnancy duration, group, parity and sex. The stars indicate significant total model p-values of the (final) multivariable-adjusted analysis (F-test, ANCOVA, * $p < 0.05$, ** $p \leq 0.01$, *** $p \leq 0.001$) and in the Spearman correlation coefficient in the analysis of the newborns.

4.3 Breast milk fatty acid profile in relation to infant body composition

The results on the breast milk fatty acid profile and its relation to infant fat mass are shown in Paper III.

4.3.1 Sample Collection

Breast milk samples were available from n=152 women at 6 weeks pp (intervention group=IG/control group=CG= 76/76) and n=120 women at 4 months pp (IG/CG= 63/57). Fatty acid profile in RBCs was measured in a subsample of 56 infants at 4 months pp (IG/CG= 29/27) and 31 infants at 12 months pp (IG/CG= 16/15).

N=188 newborns were clinically assessed at birth, n=180 infants at 6 weeks pp, n=174 infants at 4 months pp, and n=170 at 1 year of age corresponding to a drop-out rate 18%.

4.3.2 Maternal breast milk fatty acid profile over the course of lactation

Supplementation with fish oil and concomitant AA-balanced diet, starting from 15th week of gestation onwards until 4 months pp, resulted in significantly higher levels of DHA and EPA as well as higher proportions of ALA, n-3 DPA, PUFAs and total n-3 LCPUFAs in breast milk at 6 weeks pp compared to the control group (**Table 15**).

In contrast, breast milk contents of DHγLA, Adrenic acid as well as MUFA were significantly reduced in the intervention group compared to the control group at 6 weeks postpartum. Basically the same fatty acid profile was measured in breast milk taken at 4 months postpartum as shown in Table 15, demonstrating that the mothers were highly compliant to the intervention. Breast milk proportions of AA did not differ between the groups throughout lactation (**Appendix 6**).

Thus, n-3 LCPUFAs supplementation and concomitant reduction in AA intake resulted in a remarkable, significant increase in DHA and EPA contents during lactation, while the dietary intervention had no effect on AA contents in breast milk. Nevertheless, the n-6/n-3 LCPUFAs ratio was significantly reduced in the intervention group compared to the control group throughout the entire lactation period ($p<0.001$, shown in Table 15 and Appendix 6).

Table 15: Breast milk fatty acid profile

fatty acid	group	n	6th wk pp mean ± SD	n	16th wk pp mean ± SD	p‡
18:2n6, LA	C	76	10.71 ± 2.45	57	11.17 ± 2.67	0.001
	I	76	11.26 ± 3.28	63	11.19 ± 2.50	0.010
18:3n3, ALA	C	76	0.87 ± 0.31	57	0.96 ± 0.41	0.419
	I	76	1.09 ± 0.51**	63	1.02 ± 0.45	0.073
20:3n6, DHγLA	C	76	0.36 ± 0.09	57	0.30 ± 0.08	<0.001
	I	76	0.32 ± 0.08*	63	0.27 ± 0.07*	<0.001
20:4n6, AA†	C	76	0.43 ± 0.08	57	0.40 ± 0.08	0.002
	I	76	0.43 ± 0.08	63	0.40 ± 0.07	<0.001
20:5n3, EPA†	C	76	0.08 ± 0.04	57	0.07 ± 0.04	0.756
	I	76	0.18 ± 0.15***	63	0.15 ± 0.06***	0.282
22:4n6, ADA	C	76	0.10 ± 0.03	56	0.08 ± 0.02	0.001
	I	76	0.08 ± 0.02***	63	0.07 ± 0.02**	0.007
22:5n3, DPA	C	76	0.17 ± 0.06	57	0.16 ± 0.05	0.385
	I	76	0.23 ± 0.10***	63	0.21 ± 0.07***	0.125
22:6n3, DHA†	C	76	0.28 ± 0.14	57	0.24 ± 0.13	0.022
	I	76	1.34 ± 0.67***	63	1.12 ± 0.39***	0.006
AA/DHA†	C	76	1.77 ± 0.60	57	1.94 ± 0.70	0.038
	I	76	0.37 ± 0.15***	63	0.41 ± 0.22***	0.177
SAFA	C	76	44.66 ± 3.93	57	43.68 ± 4.84	0.184
	I	76	44.09 ± 5.00	63	45.49 ± 4.41	0.017
MUFA	C	76	40.42 ± 2.79	57	41.12 ± 3.89	0.115
	I	76	38.94 ± 3.75*	63	38.05 ± 3.14***	0.202
PUFA	C	76	13.68 ± 2.72	57	13.98 ± 3.00	0.522
	I	76	15.72 ± 3.67***	63	15.09 ± 2.90*	0.027
n-3 LCPUFAs	C	76	0.66 ± 0.25	57	0.59 ± 0.21	0.011
	I	76	1.94 ± 1.04***	63	1.61 ± 0.50***	0.070
n-6 LCPUFAs	C	76	1.23 ± 0.21	57	1.07 ± 0.21	<0.001
	I	76	1.22 ± 0.20	63	1.07 ± 0.18	<0.001
n-6/n-3 LCPUFAs†	C	76	2.02 ± 0.59	57	1.94 ± 0.51	0.471
	I	76	0.71 ± 0.25***	63	0.73 ± 0.25***	0.702

Data are presented as mean ± SD (n). Values for fatty acids are expressed as a percentage of the weight of the total fatty acids (% FA). Differences in fatty acid values between the groups were compared using the Mann-Whitney-U-Test (p<0.05). Changes in maternal fatty acid profile over time (‡) were determined by using the Wilcoxon-Test (p< 0.05). Values marked with stars show significant differences between groups at the same time point (Mann-Whitney-U-Test, * p< 0.05; **p<0.01, ***p<0.001) after Bonferroni-corrections. † illustrated in **Appendix 6**.

SAFA: C4:0 – C27:0
MUFA: sum of all cis-FA with one double bound
PUFA: sum of all cis-FA with two or more double bounds
n-6 LCPUFAs: C20:2n6; 20:3n6; 20:4n6; C22:2n6; C22:4n6; C22:5n6
n-3 LCPUFAs: C20:3n3; C20:4n3; 20:5n3; C21:5n3; C22:3n3; 22:5n3; 22:6n3

4.3.3 Relationship between the fatty acid composition of breast milk and maternal blood

Breast milk contents of DHA, EPA, AA, n-3 LCPUFAs, n-6 LCPUFAs as well as the AA/DHA ratio and the n-6/n-3 LCPUFAs ratio at 6 weeks pp were significantly positively correlated with their respective LCPUFAs in maternal plasma PLs at 6 weeks and 4 months pp. This relationship was also true for RBCs fatty acid, albeit to a lesser extent (**Table 16**). There was no considerable association between maternal RBCs n-6 LCPUFAs and breast milk n-6 LCPUFAs level. The maternal breast milk n-6/n-3 LCPUFAs ratio was highly correlated with the maternal erythrocyte and plasma PLs n-6/n-3 LCPUFAs ratio at 6th week pp and 4 months pp (e.g. breast milk ~maternal plasma PLs at 4 months pp: r=0.941; p<0.001).

Table 16: Correlation coefficients between breast milk LCPUFAs and the respective LCPUFAs in maternal plasma PLs and RBCs

		n	r	n	r
Plasma PLs fatty acid	AA	143	0.626***	117	0.536***
	DHA	143	0.858***	117	0.893***
	EPA	143	0.912***	117	0.850***
	AA/DHA	143	0.899***	117	0.939***
	n-3 LCPUFAs	143	0.888***	117	0.882***
	n-6 LCPUFAs	143	0.375***	117	0.271***
	n-6/n-3 LCPUFAs	143	0.923***	117	0.941***
RBCs fatty acid	AA	143	0.199*	116	0.234*
	DHA	143	0.638***	117	0.637***
	EPA	141	0.648***	117	0.628***
	AA/DHA	143	0.839***	116	0.874***
	n-3 LCPUFAs	143	0.600***	117	0.565***
	n-6 LCPUFAs	143	0.072	117	0.076
	n-6/n-3 LCPUFAs	143	0.815***	117	0.823***

Data are presented as Spearman correlation coefficients. Values marked with stars show significant correlations between the respective fatty acid in breast milk and maternal blood lipids (Spearman: *p<0.05, ***p<0.001).

4.3.4 Infant blood fatty acid profile in RBCs

Infants born to mothers of the intervention group did not significantly differ in their RBCs contents of DHA, EPA or AA at 4 months and 12 months pp when compared with the control group (**Table 17, Appendix 7**). However, the n-6/n-3 LCPUFAs ratio was significantly lower in infants of the intervention group at 4 months pp, while the AA/DHA ratio was significantly lower at both time points, at 4 and 12 months pp.

Table 17: Infant RBCs fatty acid profile

fatty acid	group	n	mean ± SD	n	mean ± SD	p‡
18:2n6, LA	C	27	5.66 ± 1.72	15	5.73 ± 2.31	0.575
	I	29	5.46 ± 1.93	16	6.88 ± 2.03	0.499
18:3n3, ALA	C	27	0.08 ± 0.04	15	0.14 ± 0.04	0.008
	I	28	0.10 ± 0.03	16	0.15 ± 0.07	0.043
20:3n6, DHγLA	C	27	1.04 ± 0.51	15	0.66 ± 0.50	0.005
	I	29	0.90 ± 0.49	16	0.76 ± 0.35	0.128
20:4n6, AA	C	27	8.76 ± 5.33	15	4.95 ± 4.23	0.007
	I	29	7.36 ± 4.98	16	6.73 ± 3.70	0.237
20:5n3, EPA	C	24	0.22 ± 0.19	15	0.11 ± 0.12	0.008
	I	29	0.37 ± 0.31	16	0.14 ± 0.10	0.063
22:4n6, ADA	C	27	1.84 ± 1.20	15	1.01 ± 0.87	0.013
	I	29	1.15 ± 0.84*	16	1.46 ± 1.06	0.499
22:5n3, DPA	C	27	0.95 ± 0.70	15	0.53 ± 0.67	0.005
	I	27	0.74 ± 0.55	16	0.72 ± 0.58	0.612
22:6n3, DHA	C	27	3.05 ± 2.42	15	1.21 ± 1.43	0.005
	I	29	4.46 ± 3.23	16	1.94 ± 1.48	0.063
AA/DHA†	C	27	3.82 ± 1.48	15	5.65 ± 1.97	0.005
	I	29	2.14 ± 0.69***	16	4.49 ± 2.01*	0.018
SAFA	C	35	56.44 ± 10.27	15	61.86 ± 9.55	0.028
	I	37	57.97 ± 11.32	16	56.73 ± 9.04	>0.99
MUFA	C	35	20.73 ± 1.83	15	22.90 ± 1.87	0.013
	I	37	20.41 ± 1.95	16	23.46 ± 2.67	0.018
PUFA	C	27	22.38 ± 11.82	15	14.84 ± 10.16	0.007
	I	29	21.11 ± 12.61	16	19.45± 9.23	0.176
n-3 LCPUFAs	C	27	4.23 ± 3.29	15	1.86 ± 2.21	0.005
	I	29	5.56 ± 4.57	16	2.83 ± 2.14	0.063
n-6 LCPUFAs	C	27	12.36 ± 7.31	15	7.06 ± 5.89	0.009
	I	29	9.95 ± 6.55	16	9.54 ± 5.32	0.237
n-6/n-3 LCPUFAs†	C	27	3.91 ± 1.54	15	5.33 ± 1.90	0.005
	I	29	2.35 ± 0.79***	16	4.29 ± 1.73	0.028

Data are presented as mean ± SD (n). Values for fatty acids are expressed as (% FA). Differences in fatty acid values between the groups were compared using the Mann-Whitney-U-Test (p<0.05). Changes in infant fatty acid profile over time (‡) were determined by using the Wilcoxon-Test (p< 0.05). Values marked with stars show significant differences between groups at the same time point (Mann-Whitney-U-Test, * p< 0.05; **p<0.01; ***p<0.001) after Bonferroni-corrections.† illustrated in **Appendix 7**.
n-6 LCPUFAs: C20:2n6; 20:3n6; 20:4n6; C22:2n6; C22:4n6; C22:5n6
n-3 LCPUFAs: C20:3n3; C20:4n3; 20:5n3; C21:5n3; C22:3n3; 22:5n3; 22:6n3

4.3.5 Relationship between the fatty acid composition of breast milk and infant RBCs

There was no significant correlation between breast milk fatty acid contents of DHA, EPA or AA at 4 months pp and their respective fatty acids in infant RBCs at 4 months and 12 months pp (**Table 18**). There was a significant positive correlation between the n-6/n-3 LCPUFAs ratio in breast milk at 4 months of lactation and the n-6/n-3 LCPUFAs ratio in infant erythrocytes at 4 months pp (n=51; r=0.505, p<0.001) and even at 12 months pp (n=29; r=0.387; p<0.05). Significant positive correlations were also found for the breast milk AA/DHA ratio at 4 months pp and infant RBCs AA/DHA ratio at 4 months (n=51; r=0.619; p<0.001) as well as 12 months pp (n=29; r=0.467; p<0.05).

Table 18: Correlation coefficients between breast milk LCPUFAs and the respective LCPUFAs in infant plasma PLs and RBCs

	Breast milk		4 months pp		12 months pp
RBCs fatty acid		N	r	n	r
	AA	51	0.020	29	-0.248
	DHA	51	0.209	29	0.300
	EPA	49	0.167	29	0.256
	AA/DHA	51	0.619***	29	0.467*
	n-3 LCPUFAs	51	0.142	29	0.204
	n-6 LCPUFAs	51	0.105	29	-0.208
	n-6/n-3 LCPUFAs	51	0.505***	29	0.387*

Data are presented as Spearman correlation coefficients. Values marked with stars show significant correlations between the respective fatty acid in breast milk and infant blood (Spearman: *p<0.05, ***p<0.001).

4.3.6 Relationship between breast milk fatty acid profile and infant growth and body composition

Potential influences of maternal breast milk fatty acid profile on infant growth and infant body composition were explored by means of multiple regression models and partial correlations. To clarify the effect of early (6th week pp) and late (4 months pp) breast milk fatty acid profile on infant outcomes, associations were performed for both time points. Results were controlled for gestational age, parity, infant sex, group, Ponderal Index at birth and breastfeeding status. The fatty acid profiles in these analyses comprise DHA, EPA, n-3 LCPUFAs, AA, n-6 LCPUFAs content in breast milk as well as AA/DHA and n-6/n-3 LCPFA ratio. Data are shown for selected fatty acids, only.

a) Early breast milk fatty acid profile (6 weeks pp) in relation to infant growth and body composition

There were significant positive associations between DHA, EPA and total n-3 LCPUFAs and different measures of infant fat mass across all time points:

DHA, EPA and total n-3 LCPUFAs in early breast milk were significantly positively associated with the sum of 4 SF at 1 year of age, and for DHA also at 4 months pp (**Table 19**).

Furthermore the n-3 fatty acids were significantly positively associated with some individual skinfolds at the different time points over the 1st y of life (data not shown): e.g., DHA, EPA and n-3 LCPUFAs in early breast milk were significantly positively related to biceps SFT in the 4-months olds (r=0.14; r=0.16; r=0.15; p<0.05), while DHA and n-3 LCPUFAs were also significantly positively related with triceps SFT in the 1-year-olds (r=0.24; r=0.25; p<0.05). Altough a trend only, there were positive associations between breast milk EPA and triceps SFT (r=0.23, p=0.054), subscapular SFT (r=0.16, p=0.09), suprailiac SFT (r=0.13, p=0.092), percentage body fat (r=0.18, p=0.056) and fat mass (g) (r=0.23, p=0.077) at 1 y pp.

Early breast milk DHA and n-3 LCPUFAs were significantly positively related to the US SC/PP ratio at 6 weeks postpartum (Table 19).

In contrast, consistent negative associations were found between AA and the total n-6 LCPUFAs and weight, Ponderal Index, BMI and LBM

(g) up to 4 months pp, as well as between AA and total n-6 LCPUFAs and fat mass (g) up to 6 weeks pp, but not at 1 y of age (**Table 20**). Early breast milk n-6 LCPUFAs were significantly negatively related to individual SFT, e.g. triceps and suprailiac SFT (r=-0.19; r=-0.17, p<0.05), the sum 4 SFT and percentage body fat at 6 weeks pp, too (r=-0.19; r=-0.18, p<0.05).

The AA/DHA ratio in early breast milk was significantly negatively related to BMI and LBM (g) at 6 weeks pp, but not at 4 months or 1 year pp. The n-6/n-3 LCPUFAs ratio in breast milk at 6 weeks pp was significantly negatively related to BMI and Ponderal Index at 6 weeks pp, and with waist circumference at 1 year pp (data not shown).

Neither the AA/DHA ratio nor the total n-6/total n-3 LCPUFAs ratio in early breast milk were significantly related to individual SFT or the sum 4 SFT from 6 weeks pp up to 1y pp (data not shown).

b) Late breast milk fatty acid profile (4 months pp) in relation to infant growth and body composition

DHA, EPA and n-3 LCPUFAs proportions in breast milk collected at 4 months pp were significantly negatively related to length at 1 year pp (e.g. EPA: ßadj -12.43 cm [95% CI -20.36, -4.231]; r= -0.13; p=0.004, n=117), and for EPA and n-3 LCPUFAs also with length at 4 months pp (e.g. EPA: ßadj -7.84 cm [95% CI -14.94, -0.73]; r= -0.12; p=0.033, n=119). Breast milk proportions of DHA, EPA and n-3 LCPUFAs at 4 months pp were significantly positively related to Ponderal Index at 1 year pp, while breast milk DHA content was significantly positively associated with BMI 1 y pp, also (e.g. Breast milk DHA at 4 mo pp ~ BMI at 1 y pp: ßadj 0.86 kg/m^2 [95% CI 0.11, 1.62]; r= -0.15; p=0.026, n=117). The AA/DHA and n-6/n-3 LCPUFAs ratio in breast milk taken at 4 months pp was significantly negatively related to the abdominal PP fat layer assessed by abdominal ultrasonography at 4 months of age (data not shown). This relationship was not observed at 6 weeks or 1 year pp.

No further significant or consistent relationships were observed between the fatty acid profile in breast milk at 4 months and infant clinical outcomes up to 1 year of age, neither for the growth indices nor for measures of fat mass assessed by SFT or ultrasound (data not shown).

Table 19: Final adjusted multiple regression analysis and partial correlation coefficients on the effect of maternal breast milk n-3 fatty acid profile at early (6th week pp) lactation on infant body composition[1]

		n	Breast milk DHA 6th week pp adj beta (95% CI)	r	Breast milk EPA 6th week pp adj beta (95% CI)	r	Breast milk n-3 LCPUFAs 6th week pp adj beta (95% CI)	r
Sum 4 SFT [mm]	6 weeks	152	0.08(-0.49, 2.11)	0.03	3.37(-2.39, 9.13)	0.08	0.50(-0.34, 1.33)	0.05
	4 months	148	1.55(0.12, 2.98)	0.12*	5.25(-1.15, 11.66)	0.11	0.90(-0.03, 1.82)	0.12
	12 months	141	1.43(0.01, 2.84)	0.16*	6.53(0.29, 12.77)	0.20*	0.91(0.00, 1.82)	0.18*
Fat mass [g]	6 weeks	152	31.89(-44.31, 108.09)	0.06	119.76(-218.36, 457.87)	0.09	17.61(-31.36, 66.58)	0.07
	4 months	147	96.49(0.57, 192.4)	0.19	252.44(-174.72, 679.60)	0.16	50.34(-11.42, 112.09)	0.18
	12 months	141	125.02(-18.4, 268.44)	0.22	575.84(-56.7, 1208.39)	0.23	78.88(-13.06, 170.81)	0.23
Body fat [%]	6 weeks	152	0.64(-0.37, 1.66)	0.02	2.72(-1.79, 7.23)	0.07	0.39(-0.26, 1.05)	0.04
	4 months	148	1.00(0.05, 1.95)	0.12*	3.29(-0.96, 7.54)	0.11	0.56(-0.05, 1.18)	0.12
	12 months	141	0.95(-0.01, 1.9)	0.16	4.16(-0.07, 8.39)	0.18	0.59(-0.03, 1.20)	0.17
US SC/PP R	6 weeks	125	0.49(0.02, 0.95)	0.10*	1.66(-0.36, 3.67)	0.12	0.30(0.01, 0.60)	0.12*
	4 months	126	0.26(-0.27, 0.78)	0.09	0.58(-1.7, 2.87)	0.06	0.16(-0.17, 0.49)	0.09
	12 months	132	0.11(-0.14, 0.36)	0.04	0.66(-0.43, 1.75)	0.10	0.08(-0.08, 0.24)	0.06

[1] Data are presented as the regression coefficient of the fatty acid of interest (beta) along with the (95% confidence interval) and the partial correlation coefficient according to Spearman (r) of the fatty acid of interest. The stars indicate significant total model p-values of the (final) multivariable-adjusted analysis (F-test, ANCOVA) and in the Spearman correlation coefficient (*p< 0.05; **p<0.01).

Table 20: Final adjusted multiple regression analysis and partial correlation coefficients on the effect of maternal breast milk n-6 fatty acid profile at early lactation (6th week pp) on infant growth and growth indices over the 1st year of life [1]

		n	Breast milk AA 6th week pp		Breast milk n-6 LCPUFAs 6th week pp	
			adj beta (95% CI)	r	adj beta (95% CI)	r
Weight [g]	6 weeks	152	-1833.53 (-2926.5, -740.56)	-0.32**	-779.34 (-1201.38, -357.3)	-0.36***
	4 months	148	-1608.45 (-2978.68, -238.22)	-0.23*	-687.65 (-1218.36, -156.95)	-0.26*
	12 months	146	-1410.28 (-3447.83, 627.42)	-0.13	-261.16 (-1060.42, 538.10)	-0.06
Length [g]	6 weeks	152	-1.92 (-6.19, 2.35)	-0.11	-0.55 (-2.21, 1.12)	-0.12
	4 months	149	-0.09 (-4.29, 4.11)	0.05	-0.26 (-1.9, 1.37)	-0.09
	12 months	146	-0.97 (-6.32, 4.38)	-0.01	0.11 (-1.98, 2.20)	0.03
BMI [kg/m²]	6 weeks	152	-4.88 (-7.32, -2.44)	-0.35***	-2.23 (-3.16, -1.3)	-0.41***
	4 months	148	-4.08 (-6.81, -1.35)	-0.25**	-1.65 (-2.71, -0.59)	-0.27**
	12 months	146	-1.93 (-4.67, 0.82)	-0.16	-0.52 (-1.60, 0.55)	-0.11
PI [kg/m³]	6 weeks	152	-7.60 (-12.81, -2.40)	-0.26**	-3.70 (-5.70, -1.71)	-0.31***
	4 months	148	-6.62 (-11.42, -1.83)	-0.23**	-2.46 (-4.32, -0.59)	-0.22*
	12 months	146	-2.08 (-6.14, 1.98)	-0.13	-0.67 (-2.26, 0.91)	-0.10
LBM [g]	6 weeks	152	-1278.53 (-2017.73, -539.33)	-0.33**	-511.42 (-798.30, -224.55)	-0.36**
	4 months	147	-1057.03 (-2004.02, -110.04)	-0.23*	-491.69 (-857.20, -126.18)	-0.29**
	12 months	141	-1002.19 (-2394.59, 390.20)	-0.12	-141.72 (-686.50, 403.05)	-0.05

[1] Data are presented as the regression coefficient of the fatty acid of interest (beta) along with the (95% confidence interval) and the partial correlation coefficient according to Spearman (r) of the fatty acid of interest. The stars indicate significant total model p-values of the (final) multivariable-adjusted analysis (F-test, ANCOVA) and in the Spearman correlation coefficient (*p< 0.05; **p<0.01; ***p<0.001).

4.4 Sonographic assessment of infant body composition in relation to anthropometry and skinfold thickness measurement

Sonographic assessment of subcutaneous and preperitoneatal fat mass was performed in 160 infants 6 weeks after birth (n=76 girls vs. n=84 boys) and in 158 children at 4 months of age (n=78 girls vs. n=80 boys). 156 infants completed the ultrasound investigations at 1 y of age (n=81 girls vs. n=75 boys) (Paper IV).

4.4.1 Precision of ultrasonography

To calculate error of precision, three complete investigations of n=12 infants (n=4 out of each age group) were used. In each case three images in the axial plane and three images in the sagittal plane, thus 18 images per child, were evaluated by a pediatrician (E.H.). The results from precision measuring are shown as error of precision (EP_{RMS}) and as Intraclass-correlation-coefficient (ICC) in **Table 21** and **22**.

Table 21: Error of precision, shown as EP$_{RMS}$ in % of fat thicknesses measured and as areas for all infants in their age group, respectively.

		All	6 wk	4 mo	1 y
Individual (i) measurements	sag$_i$ cranial pp	11.0%	10.4%	13.0%	9.2%
	sag$_i$ caudal pp	21.1%	21.6%	22.4%	19.2%
	sag$_i$ cranial sc	6.8%	7.6%	7.1%	5.4%
	sag$_i$ caudal sc	8.0%	10.2%	6.9%	6.5%
	ax$_i$ r	10.0%	12.3%	8.7%	8.6%
	ax$_i$ m	9.5%	12.0%	8.5%	7.3%
	ax$_i$ l	10.1%	11.9%	9.5%	8.6%
Mean out of 3 measurements	sag cranial pp	6.7%	7.4%	6.8%	5.8%
	sag caudal pp	13.9%	14.9%	15.5%	10.5%
	sag cranial sc	4.6%	5.8%	3.8%	3.8%
	sag caudal sc	5.2%	7.2%	4.2%	3.2%
	ax r	6.8%	8.4%	6.5%	5.2%
	ax m	6.8%	8.9%	6.0%	4.7%
	ax l	6.2%	8.7%	5.8%	2.6%
Area	Asag pp	7.3%	8.8%	7.7%	4.8%
	Asag sc	4.5%	6.3%	3.6%	2.6%
	Aax sc	5.5%	7.2%	5.5%	2.7%

In case of individual measurements the values are based on the coefficient of variation of the nine measurements; in case of mean and areas the values are based on the coefficient of variation of three repeated measurements, respectively.

Both methods of evaluation showed the same trend, although smaller differences were better identified by the EP$_{RMS}$ method. The error of precision was reduced by averaging the three individual measurements and was further reduced by the calculation of the area, e.g. for the axial determination of subcutaneous fat EP$_{RMS}$ was reduced from 9.5% to 6.8% by average determination and again reduced to 5.5% in case of area calculation. When stratified by age group virtually all parameters showed a reduction in the error of precision.

		All	6 wk	4 mo	1 y
Individual (i) measurements	sag$_i$ cranial pp	0.86	0.86	0.87	0.74
	sag$_i$ caudal pp	0.74	0.70	0.54	0.87
	sag$_i$ cranial sc	0.97	0.89	0.97	0.98
	sag$_i$ caudal sc	0.97	0.80	0.97	0.99
	ax$_i$ r	0.95	0.77	0.96	0.95
	ax$_i$ m	0.97	0.80	0.98	0.97
	ax$_i$ l	0.95	0.75	0.96	0.96
Mean out of 3 measurements	sag cranial pp	0.93	0.94	0.94	0.83
	sag caudal pp	0.86	0.88	0.71	0.93
	sag cranial sc	0.99	0.93	0.99	0.99
	sag caudal sc	0.99	0.92	0.99	0.99
	ax r	0.98	0.92	0.98	0.98
	ax m	0.99	0.92	0.99	0.99
	ax l	0.98	0.85	0.99	0.99
Area	Asag pp	0.93	0.95	0.94	0.93
	Asag sc	0.99	0.98	0.99	0.99
	Aax sc	0.99	0.94	0.99	0.99

Table 22: Intraclass-correlation-coefficients (ICC) of the precision measurements for all infants in each age group. In case of individual measurements the values are based on the coefficient of variation of the nine measurements; in case of mean and areas the values are based on the coefficient of variation of three repeated measurements, respectively.

To compare two different observers (E.H. and D.M.) n=45 infants (n=15 out of each age group) were evaluated. In each case three sagittal and three axial pictures were evaluated. The Bland-Altman-Plots did not show any relevant differences between the observers. In the plots of all parameters the differences remained lower than ± 2 SD. The differences between the observers based on the mean of each measurement are shown in **Table 23**. The measurement of A sag pp produced the smallest error between the two observers.

		Individual (i) measurements	Mean out of 3 measurements
Individual (i)	sag$_i$ cranial pp	10.0%	5.5%
	sag$_i$ caudal pp	12.5%	9.4%
	sag$_i$ cranial sc	11.0%	8.7%
	sag$_i$ caudal sc	12.6%	8.8%
	ax$_i$ r	11.1%	8.9%
	ax$_i$ m	11.6%	9.9%
	ax$_i$ l	10.7%	8.9%
Area	Asag pp		4.3%
	Asag sc		8.1%
	Aax sc		8.4%

Table 23: Percentage interobserver-difference shown as EP$_{RMS}$ in % of average fat thicknesses and areas (n=45 infants)

4.4.2 Adipose tissue growth by age and group

Average weight of the infants was 3443 g at birth, 4764 g at 6 weeks pp, 6390 g at 4 months pp, and 9517g at 12 months pp, accounting for a BMI of 12.8 kg/m^2 at birth, 15.3 kg/m^2 at 6 weeks pp, 16.3 kg/m^2 at 4 months pp and 16.8 kg/m^2, at 12 mo pp respectively (**Table 24**, Figure 18). Weight and length as well as BMI significantly increased during the first year of life, although the increase in BMI was low from 4 months up to 1 year of age.

The skinfold thicknesses at all four body sites were significantly higher at 4 months pp compared to 3-5 days pp ($p<0.001$), and 6 weeks pp ($p<0.001$; except subscapular SFT $p>0.05$). The highest values were observed at the triceps SFT (7.8 mm) at all 4 time points. The highest increase was observed at the suprailiac SFT (6 wk pp vs. 4 mo pp: 1.1 mm; from 4.8 mm to 5.9 mm). At age 1 y, the suprailiac SFT was significantly reduced compared to 4 months pp to an average of 4.5 mm (p < 0.001). All other SFT showed similar values and were not significantly different compared to 4 months pp (Table 24).

The ultrasound investigations showed pronounced differences in the physiological growth of SC and PP fat depots over the first year of life: Thickness of SC fat layers significantly increased from 6 weeks pp (A ax sc= 30.5 mm^2) to 4 months pp (A ax sc= 44.9 mm^2) just to decrease until the first year (Aax sc= 31.5 mm^2). In contrast the PP fat layer continuously increased over time with an average A sag pp of 10.7 mm^2 in the 6-week olds, 13.1 mm^2 in the 4-months and 17.9 mm^2 in the 1y-olds (**Table 25**). Therefore, the ratio (Ratio SC/PP ratio) between the two adipose tissue compartments significantly increased from week 6 to month 4 pp (Ratio SC/PP= 3.0 versus 3.6) and decreased then until 12 months pp (Ratio = 1.7 p < 0.01). Nevertheless, subcutaneous adipose tissue had a clear predominance compared to preperitoneal fat mass, at all 3 time points of investigation.

Corresponding to the skinfold dataset, we observed no significant differences between the two dietary groups in any parameter of SC fat investigated by ultrasound (p > 0.1, Table 6). Adipose tissue development of both SC and PP fat mass had the same temporal pattern in intervention and control group (Table 6) over the first year of life as illustrated in Figure 21.

4.4.3 Differences in adipose tissue growth in boys and girls

At delivery, there were no significant differences between boys and girls in weight, length, BMI or lean body mass (Table 24). In contrast, there were sex specific differences at the following time points: At 6 weeks pp, 4 months pp and 1 year pp boys had a significantly higher body weight, length, and lean body mass compared to the girls. The boys were on average 259 g heavier at 6 weeks pp, 470 g at 4 months and 589 g at 12 months pp (p<0.001). BMI was higher in boys at 4 months pp (0.49 kg/m^2) and 12 months pp (0.48 kg/m^2) compared to the girls, respectively (Table 24). This was due to increased lean body mass (Table 24).

Of note, the girls had a significantly higher subcutaneous fat mass, assessed by a higher suprailiac SFT at 6 weeks and 4 months pp, as well as by a higher subscapular SFT at 4 months pp (Table 24). The other individual SFT measures showed no significant sex specific differences (p > 0.05).

In the sonographic evaluation, girls had a significantly higher subcutaneous fat mass compared to the boys as evidenced by higher A sag sc, A ax sc and higher individual SC distances (all p<0.001; **Table 25**), in analyses corrected for the specific time point of assessment, current body weight and length. Interestingly, there were no sex specific differences in PP fat thickness between boys and girls (Table 25).

The fat distribution was shifted towards a more centralized pattern in the girls compared to the boys: the subscapular-to-triceps SFT ratio, an index of central to peripheral fat distribution, was significantly higher in the girls at 6 weeks pp, 4 months pp and 12 months pp. Also, a higher central-to-total SFT ratio was found in girls at birth, 6 weeks, 4 months and 12 months pp compared to the boys (Table 24). The SC/PP ratio calculated based on the sonographic measurements was significantly higher in the girls compared to the boys at 6 weeks and 12 months pp (p<0.01) but not at 4 months pp (Table 25).

Table 24: Sex differences in anthropometry and adipose tissue growth assessed by SFT investigations

	parameter	All mean (SD)	n	female mean (SD)	n	male mean (SD)	n	unadjusted beta (lower, upper)
Birth	Birth weight [g]	3443.4 (520.0)	188	3369.3 (521.2)	90	3511.5 (512.2)	98	142.157 (-5.646, 289.96)
	Length at birth [cm]	51.7 (2.5)	188	51.4 (2.5)	90	51.9 (2.4)	98	0.474 (-0.239, 1.187)
	Ponderal Index [kg/m³]	24.8 (2.4)	188	24.6 (2.2)	90	25.03 (2.6)	98	0.470 (-0.218, 1.158)
	BMI at birth [kg/m²]	12.82 (1.29)	188	12.66 (1.27)	90	12.97 (1.29)	98	0.314 (-0.053, 0.68)
	Biceps SFT [mm]	3.5 (0.6)	168	3.4 (0.6)	80	3.5 (0.7)	88	0.094 (-0.101, 0.288)
	Triceps SFT [mm]	4.7 (0.9)	168	4.8 (0.9)	80	4.7 (0.9)	88	-0.072 (-0.34, 0.196)
	Subscapular SFT [mm]	4.5 (1.0)	168	4.6 (1.0)	80	4.4 (1.0)	88	-0.192 (-0.482, 0.097)
	Suprailiacal SFT [mm]	3.3 (0.7)	168	3.4 (0.8)	80	3.2 (0.6)	88	-0.207 (-0.417, 0.003)
	Sum 4 SFT [mm]	16.0 (2.6)	168	16.2 (2.5)	80	15.8 (2.8)	88	-0.377 (-1.169, 0.414)
	Body fat [%]	13.8 (2.7)	168	14.0 (2.7)	80	13.6 (2.8)	88	-0.421 (-1.245, 0.403)
	Fat mass [g]	487.5 (143.0)	168	483.9 (133.6)	80	490.7 (151.7)	88	6.820 (-36.588, 50.228)
	Lean body mass [g]	2988.7 (355.3)	168	2918.5 (339.2)	80	3052.5 (359.5)	88	133.987 (28.031, 239.943)*
	Subscapular-Triceps ratio	0.97 (0.17)	168	0.98 (0.16)	80	0.96 (0.18)	88	-0.023 (-0.074, 0.027)
	Central-to-total-SFT	48.7 (3.3)	168	49.35 (3.15)	80	48.04 (3.32)	88	-1.310 (-2.29, -0.329)**
6 wk	Weight [g]	4764.2 (614.5)	180	4628.8 (562.1)	86	4888 (636.8)	94	259.209 (83.06, 435.359)**
	Length [cm]	55.8 (2.3)	180	55.3 (2.1)	86	56.3 (2.4)	94	0.950 (0.288, 1.611)**
	Ponderal Index [kg/m³]	27.4 (2.6)	180	27.3 (2.7)	86	27.5 (2.5)	94	0.213 (-0.538, 0.964)
	BMI [kg/m²]	15.25 (1.29)	180	15.1 (1.3)	86	15.38 (1.25)	94	0.283 (-0.093, 0.659)
	Biceps SFT [mm]	4.4 (0.9)	180	4.2 (0.8)	86	4.5 (1.0)	94	0.289 (0.03, 0.547)*
	Triceps SFT [mm]	6.7 (1.4)	180	6.6 (1.3)	86	6.7 (1.4)	94	0.113 (-0.294, 0.52)
	Subscapular SFT [mm]	6.2 (1.3)	180	6.4 (1.3)	86	6.1 (1.2)	94	-0.279 (-0.644, 0.087)
	Suprailiacal SFT [mm]	4.8 (1.1)	180	5.0 (1.1)	86	4.6 (0.95)	94	-0.476 (-0.775, -0.176)**
	Sum 4 SFT [mm]	22.1 (3.78)	180	22.3 (3.6)	86	21.9 (3.9)	94	-0.353 (-1.458, 0.752)
	Body fat [%]	19.0 (3.0)	180	19.2 (2.8)	86	18.9 (3.18)	94	-0.326 (-1.207, 0.554)
	Fat mass [g]	916.2 (227.9)	180	896.6 (213.2)	86	934.1 (240.3)	94	37.542 (-29.076, 104.16)
	Lean body mass [g]	3848.0 (434.3)	180	3732.2 (393.1)	86	3953.9 (445.1)	94	221.667 (98.53, 344.804)***
	Subscapular-Triceps ratio	1.0 (0.16)	180	0.98 (0.18)	86	0.92 (0.16)	94	-0.060 (-0.109, -0.011)*
	Central-to-total-SFT	49.8 (3.5)	180	51.17 (3.33)	86	48.63 (3.26)	94	-2.538 (-3.5, -1.575)***
4 mo	Weight [g]	6389.8 (705.2)	174	6146.7 (642.0)	84	6616.6 (688.8)	90	469.910 (271.687, 668.132)***
	Length [cm]	62.5 (2.1)	175	61.7 (2.0)	85	63.2 (2.0)	90	1.409 (0.82, 1.998)***
	Ponderal Index [kg/m³]	26.1 (2.3)	174	25.97 (2.4)	84	26.3 (2.3)	90	0.281 (-0.411, 0.973)
	BMI [kg/m²]	16.3 (1.4)	174	16.1 (1.3)	84	16.6 (1.35)	90	0.491 (0.095, 0.887)*
	Biceps SFT [mm]	5.085 (1.0)	174	5.1 (1.1)	84	5.1 (0.9)	90	0.040 (-0.249, 0.329)
	Triceps SFT [mm]	7.748 (1.5)	174	7.8 (1.6)	84	7.7 (1.4)	90	-0.018 (-0.467, 0.431)
	Subscapular SFT [mm]	6.46 (1.3)	174	6.7 (1.4)	84	6.27 (1.1)	90	-0.393 (-0.777, -0.009)*
	Suprailiacal SFT [mm]	5.938 (1.4)	174	6.3 (1.6)	84	5.6 (1.2)	90	-0.700 (-1.117, -0.283)**
	Sum 4 SFT [mm]	25.23 (4.1)	174	25.8 (4.6)	84	24.7 (3.7)	90	-1.071 (-2.297, 0.155)
	Body fat [%]	21.09 (2.8)	174	21.4 (3.0)	84	20.8 (2.5)	90	-0.658 (-1.472, 0.157)
	Fat mass [g]	1354.8 (274.5)	173	1324.4 (279.1)	83	1382.9 (268.7)	90	58.515 (-23.127, 140.156)
	Lean body mass [g]	5031.6 (513.0)	173	4812.4 (451.4)	83	5233.7 (484.5)	90	421.314 (281.45, 561.179)***
	Subscapular-Triceps ratio	0.9 (0.2)	174	0.88 (0.21)	84	0.82 (0.15)	90	-0.061 (-0.115, -0.007)*
	Central-to-total-SFT	49.0 (4.5)	174	50.20 (4.38)	84	47.97 (3.39)	90	-2.228 (-3.387, -1.068)***
12 mo	Weight [g]	9517.4 (1035.8)	170	9219.6 (950.1)	84	9808.2 (1038.5)	86	588.614 (289.195, 888.032)***
	Length [cm]	75.2 (2.6)	170	74.6 (2.7)	84	75.8 (2.4)	86	1.187 (0.422, 1.952)**
	Ponderal Index [kg/m³]	22.4 (2.1)	170	22.2 (2.3)	84	22.5 (1.9)	86	0.271 (-0.349, 0.89)
	BMI [kg/m²]	16.80 (1.42)	170	16.6 (1.46)	84	17.04 (1.35)	86	0.484 (0.062, 0.905)*
	Biceps SFT [mm]	5.2 (1.2)	169	5.3 (1.4)	83	5.1 (1.1)	86	-0.275 (-0.649, 0.099)
	Triceps SFT [mm]	7.94 (1.6)	169	7.8 (1.4)	83	8.1 (1.8)	86	0.257 (-0.236, 0.75)
	Subscapular SFT [mm]	6.4 (1.4)	170	6.5 (1.4)	84	6.3 (1.3)	86	-0.244 (-0.653, 0.165)
	Suprailiacal SFT [mm]	4.5 (1.0)	165	4.7 (1.1)	80	4.3 (0.9)	85	-0.372 (-0.68, -0.064)*
	Sum 4 SFT [mm]	24.1 (4.2)	165	24.4 (4.4)	80	23.7 (4.0)	85	-0.705 (-1.995, 0.585)
	Body fat [%]	19.7 (2.9)	165	19.95 (2.97)	80	19.5 (2.8)	85	-0.461 (-1.339, 0.418)
	Fat mass [g]	1894.4 (429.9)	165	1857.2 (414.7)	80	1929.3 (443.3)	85	72.091 (-59.09, 203.272)
	Lean body mass [g]	7637.6 (714.9)	165	7385.1 (656.4)	80	7875.1 (689.0)	85	490.007 (284.409, 695.605)***
	Subscapular-Triceps ratio	0.8 (0.2)	169	0.84 (0.15)	83	0.79 (0.17)	86	-0.047 (-0.096, 0.002)
	Central-to-total-SFT	45.3 (3.9)	165	45.88 (3.39)	80	44.66 (4.21)	85	-1.221 (-2.392, -0.05)*

Data are presented as mean ± SD (n) along with the non-adjusted mean difference (95% confidence interval). Values marked with stars show significant differences between groups (Student's t-test, *p<0.05; **p<0.01; ***p<0.001).

Table 25: Sex differences in adipose tissue growth and fat distribution assessed by ultrasonography

	parameter	All mean (SD)	n	female mean (SD)	n	male mean (SD)	n	unadjusted beta	(lower, upper)	adjusted beta adj.	(lower, upper)
6 weeks	sag$_i$ cranial sc [mm]	3.08 (1.24)	158	3.33 (1.22)	75	2.85 (1.22)	83	-0.48	(-0.86, -0.1)*	-0.76	(-1.06, -0.45)***
	sag$_i$ caudal sc [mm]	3.09 (1.24)	158	3.29 (1.18)	75	2.91 (1.28)	83	-0.38	(-0.76, 0.01)	-0.65	(-0.97, -0.34)***
	sag$_i$ cranial pp [mm]	1.42 (0.43)	150	1.39 (0.42)	71	1.44 (0.44)	79	0.05	(-0.09, 0.19)	0.01	(-0.13, 0.15)
	sag$_i$ caudal pp [mm]	0.74 (0.46)	150	0.80 (0.57)	71	0.68 (0.31)	79	-0.12	(-0.26, 0.03)	-0.13	(-0.28, 0.02)
	ax$_i$r [mm]	3.11 (1.25)	160	3.25 (1.15)	76	2.98 (1.33)	84	-0.27	(-0.66, 0.11)	-0.57	(-0.88, -0.25)***
	ax$_i$m [mm]	3.02 (1.27)	160	3.20 (1.20)	76	2.86 (1.32)	84	-0.34	(-0.73, 0.05)	-0.64	(-0.96, -0.33)***
	ax$_i$l [mm]	3.06 (1.26)	160	3.21 (1.18)	76	2.93 (1.32)	84	-0.28	(-0.67, 0.11)	-0.58	(-0.89, -0.26)***
	Aax sc [mm^2]	30.5 (12.5)	160	32.2 (11.7)	76	29.0 (13.1)	84	-3.1	(-7.0, 0.7)	-6.2	(-9.2, -3.1)***
	Asag sc [mm^2]	30.8 (12.4)	158	33.1 (11.9)	75	28.8 (12.4)	83	-4.4	(-8.2, -0.6)*	-7.1	(-10.2, -4.0)***
	Asag pp [mm^2]	10.7 (3.7)	152	10.8 (4.1)	72	10.5 (3.4)	80	-0.3	(-1.5, 0.9)	-0.5	(-1.7, 0.7)
	R SC/PP	3.04 (1.35)	150	3.21 (1.23)	71	2.89 (1.44)	79	-0.33	(-0.76, 0.10)	-0.55	(-0.93, -0.17)***
4 months	sag$_i$ cranial sc [mm]	4.11 (1.51)	155	4.39 (1.49)	76	3.85 (1.50)	79	-0.54	(-1.01, -0.07)*	-0.98	(-1.39, -0.57)***
	sag$_i$ caudal sc [mm]	4.18 (1.52)	155	4.43 (1.50)	76	3.95 (1.50)	79	-0.48	(-0.95, -0.01)*	-0.89	(-1.31, -0.47)***
	sag$_i$ cranial pp [mm]	1.78 (0.59)	148	1.85 (0.58)	73	1.71 (0.59)	75	-0.14	(-0.33, 0.05)	-0.21	(-0.41, -0.02)*
	sag$_i$ caudal pp [mm]	0.85 (0.36)	148	0.85 (0.33)	73	0.86 (0.38)	75	0.01	(-0.10, 0.13)	-0.02	(-0.14, 0.1)
	ax$_i$r [mm]	4.54 (1.66)	158	4.84 (1.69)	78	4.24 (1.58)	80	-0.60	(-1.11, -0.09)*	-1.08	(-1.53, -0.64)***
	ax$_i$m [mm]	4.43 (1.69)	158	4.77 (1.78)	78	4.1 (1.55)	80	-0.68	(-1.19, -0.16)*	-1.17	(-1.62, -0.71)***
	ax$_i$l [mm]	4.54 (1.66)	158	4.84 (1.73)	78	4.25 (1.55)	80	-0.59	(-1.10, -0.08)*	-1.05	(-1.50, -0.60)***
	Aax sc [mm^2]	44.9 (16.6)	158	48.2 (17.2)	78	41.7 (15.4)	80	-6.5	(-11.5, -1.4)*	-11.2	(-15.7, -6.8)***
	Asag sc [mm^2]	41.5 (15.1)	155	44.1 (14.9)	76	39.0 (14.9)	79	-5.1	(-9.8, -0.4)*	-9.4	(-13.5, -5.2)***
	Asag pp [mm^2]	13.1 (4.1)	148	13.4 (3.8)	73	12.7 (4.3)	75	-0.7	(-2.0, 0.6)	-1.2	(-2.6, 0.1)
	R SC/PP	3.60 (1.48)	148	3.73 (1.56)	73	3.47 (1.39)	75	-0.26	(-0.73, 0.22)	-0.50	(-0.99, 0.00)
12 months	sag$_i$ cranial sc [mm]	2.79 (1.3)	154	2.96 (1.39)	79	2.61 (1.18)	75	-0.35	(-0.76, 0.06)	-0.71	(-1.04, -0.38)***
	sag$_i$ caudal sc [mm]	2.9 (1.37)	154	3.08 (1.5)	79	2.70 (1.2)	75	-0.38	(-0.81, 0.05)	-0.73	(-1.09, -0.38)***
	sag$_i$ cranial pp [mm]	2.36 (0.71)	153	2.39 (0.68)	78	2.33 (0.74)	75	-0.06	(-0.28, 0.17)	-0.17	(-0.39, 0.06)
	sag$_i$ caudal pp [mm]	1.22 (0.55)	153	1.23 (0.57)	78	1.21 (0.53)	75	-0.01	(-0.19, 0.16)	-0.08	(-0.26, 0.1)
	ax$_i$r [mm]	3.19 (1.55)	156	3.42 (1.74)	81	2.95 (1.28)	75	-0.47	(-0.95, 0.01)	-0.83	(-1.26, -0.41)***
	ax$_i$m [mm]	3.13 (1.57)	156	3.39 (1.76)	81	2.86 (1.28)	75	-0.53	(-1.01, -0.04)*	-0.87	(-1.30, -0.43)***
	ax$_i$l [mm]	3.16 (1.51)	156	3.37 (1.7)	81	2.93 (1.24)	75	-0.44	(-0.91, 0.03)	-0.78	(-1.19, -0.37)***
	Aax sc [mm^2]	31.5 (15.4)	156	33.9 (17.3)	81	29. (12.7)	75	-4.9	(-9.7, -0.1)*	-8.4	(-12.6, -4.1)***
	Asag sc [mm^2]	28.4 (13.3)	154	30.1 (14.4)	79	26.6 (11.8)	75	-3.5	(-7.7, 0.7)	-7.1	(-10.5, -3.6)***
	Asag pp [mm^2]	17.9 (5.8)	153	18.1 (5.9)	78	17.7 (5.7)	75	-0.4	(-2.2, 1.5)	-1.2	(-3.1, 0.6)
	R SC/PP	1.74 (0.78)	151	1.83 (0.79)	76	1.64 (0.72)	75	-0.18	(-0.42, 0.06)	-0.31	(-0.53, -0.09)**

Data are presented as mean ± SD (n) along with the non-adjusted mean difference (95% confidence interval). The last column gives the adjusted mean difference (95% CI) from multiple regression analysis (F-test, ANCOVA) controlling for age, current weight and length. Values marked with stars show significant differences between groups (Student´s t-test, *p<0.05; **p<0.01; ***p<0.001).

4.4.4 Correlation coefficients of the different measures of fat mass

Body weight was significantly correlated with the anthropometric and sonographic fat measurements at all three time points. The highest correlation was observed between body weight and the suprailiac SFT (r=0.53), and between body weight and A ax sc (r=0.56) and A sag sc (r=0.54) at 6 weeks postpartum (**Table 26**). Subcutaneous fat was more highly correlated with weight than preperitoneal fat at all time points (e.g. at 6 weeks pp: weight vs. Aax sc with r = 0.56 and App with r= 0.17, Table 26). Likewise, BMI was more highly correlated with measures of subcutaneous fat compared to preperitoneal fat tissue (e.g. 6 weeks pp: BMI vs. Aax sc with r=0.60 and App n.s. Table 26).

Table 26: Spearman-correlation-coefficients for anthropometric measures

6 weeks	weight	length	BMI
Biceps SFT	0.41	0.22	0.43
Triceps SFT	0.42	0.21	0.45
Subscapular SFT	**0.50**	0.21	**0.54**
Suprailiac SFT	**0.53**	0.21	**0.61**
Asag pp	0.17	n.s.	n.s. †
Aax sc	**0.56**	0.26	**0.60**
Asag sc	**0.54**	0.27	**0.57**†
R sc/pp	0.44	0.24	0.45†
4 months	**weight**	**length**	**BMI**
Biceps SFT	0.24	n.s.	0.30
Triceps SFT	0.31	n.s.	0.37
Subscapular SFT	**0.36**	n.s.	**0.46**
Suprailiac SFT	**0.33**	n.s.	**0.46**
Asag pp	n.s.	n.s.	0.20†
Aax sc	**0.42**	n.s.	**0.51**
Asag sc	**0.39**	n.s.	**0.48**†
R sc/pp	n.s.	n.s.	0.27†
1 year	**weight**	**length**	**BMI**
Biceps SFT	0.28	n.s.	0.42
Triceps SFT	0.44	n.s.	0.51
Subscapular SFT	**0.49**	n.s.	**0.60**
Suprailiac SFT	0.36	n.s.	0.47
Asag pp	0.24	n.s.	0.27†
Aax sc	**0.40**	n.s.	**0.55**
Asag sc	**0.44**	n.s.	**0.57**†
R sc/pp	0.44	n.s.	0.44†

† shown in **Figure 22**; n=180 at 6 weeks pp, n=174 at 4 months pp, n=165 at 12 months pp; numbers in bold face demonstrate the highest correlation coefficients, n.s. non significant

Table 27: Spearman-correlation coefficients of the sonographic measures

6 weeks	Asag pp	Asag sc	Aax sc	R sc/pp
Asag sc	0.23†			
Aax sc	0.24	0.92		
R sc/pp	-0.42	0.72	0.72	
sag cranial pp	**0.85**	0.21	0.23	-0.35
sag caudal pp	**0.77**	0.21	0.22	-0.30
sag cranial sc	0.23	**0.99**	0.90	0.71
sag caudal sc	0.23	**0.99**	0.92	0.73
ax r	0.23	0.90	**0.98**	0.71
ax m	0.25	0.90	**0.99**	0.70
ax l	0.22	0.89	**0.98**	0.72
4 months	**Asag pp**	**Asag sc**	**Aax sc**	**R sc/pp**
Asag sc	0.23†			
Aax sc	0.26	0.90		
R sc/pp	-0.53	0.64	0.61	
sag cranial pp	**0.90**	0.26	0.25	-0.45
sag caudal pp	**0.74**	n.s.	0.21	-0.41
sag cranial sc	0.22	**0.99**	0.90	0.65
sag caudal sc	0.24	**0.99**	0.90	0.62
ax r	0.24	0.89	**0.98**	0.62
ax m	0.28	0.90	**0.99**	0.60
ax l	0.26	0.88	**0.97**	0.60
1 year	**Asag pp**	**Asag sc**	**Aax sc**	**R sc/pp**
Asag sc	0.49†			
Aax sc	0.49	0.92		
R sc/pp	-0.18	0.72	0.72	
sag cranial pp	**0.94**	0.44	0.43	-0.19
sag caudal pp	**0.89**	0.47	0.47	n.s.
sag cranial sc	0.47	**0.99**	0.90	0.72
sag caudal sc	0.51	**0.99**	0.93	0.71
ax r	0.47	0.91	**0.99**	0.72
ax m	0.49	0.92	**1.00**	0.71
ax l	0.48	0.91	**0.99**	0.70

† shown in **Figure 22**; n=152 at 6 weeks pp, n=155 at 4 months pp, n=153 at 12 months p, numbers in bold face demonstrate the highest correlation coefficients, n.s. non significant

The correlation coefficients of the sonographic measures showed very high correlation coefficients for the different measures of subcutaneous fat among each other (r > 0.9). This was also true for preperitoneal fat (r>0.74). The correlations between preperitoneal and subcutaneous adipose tissue were weak (r < 0.24) at 6 weeks, underlining the independency of both fat depots (**Table 27**), but became stronger with increasing age (r < 0.50). The ratio of subcutaneous to preperitoneal fat was more highly correlated with subcutaneous fat (r = 0.72 vs. r = -0.42), which results from the high variability of the latter (Table 27). Similar results were obtained when the analysis was corrected for the effects of group, sex and the age at the investigation (data not shown).

The correlation-coefficients between the fat tissue assessed by anthropometry and ultrasonography demonstrated the co-existence of different independent fat depots (**Table 28**). The sonographic assessment of preperitoneal fat tissue demonstrated very weak correlations with all other fat measures, especially at 6 weeks and 4 months pp (r < 0.25) and, therefore, was considered as an independent parameter, which showed moderate correlations with the sum 4 SFT, the subscapular and suprailiac SFT at 12 month pp, only (r < 0.42). In contrast, the sonographic measures of SC fat tissue were highly correlated with the sum SFT at 6 weeks, 4 months and especially at 12 months pp (range: r=0.62-0.71; Table 28), the subscapular (r = 0.70) and the suprailiac SFT (r=0.68) and therefore reflect another compartment. SFT measurement at biceps, triceps and arm circumference showed moderate correlations among each other (r ~ 0.45) and towards the other measurements, except PP fat (e.g. r < 0.24 at 12 months pp). The partial correlation analyses corrected for group, sex and age at the investigation revealed similar results (data not shown).

Table 28: Spearman-correlation coefficients of the different fat measures

6 weeks	Biceps	Triceps	Sub-scapular	Supra-iliac	BMI	Asag pp	Asag sc	Aax sc	R sc/pp
PI	0.32	0.34	0.43	0.47	0.88	n.s.	0.41	0.45	0.32
Armcircumf.	0.46	0.53	0.48	0.57	0.71	0.17	0.54	0.53	0.38
Biceps		0.62	0.49	0.47	0.43	0.18	0.39	0.35	0.24
Triceps			0.62	0.55	0.45	0.17	0.51	0.50	0.33
Subscapular				0.52	0.54	n.s.	0.60	0.65	0.50
Suprailiac					0.61	0.23	0.65	0.63	0.47
Sum 4 SFT					0.61	0.20†	0.66†	0.65	0.46
4 months	Biceps	Triceps	Sub-scapular	Supra-iliac	BMI	A pp	Asag sc	Aax sc	R sc/pp
PI	0.27	0.35	0.43	0.45	0.92	0.23	0.46	0.48	0.21
Armcircumf.	0.43	0.40	0.42	0.43	0.68	n.s.	0.40	0.47	0.28
Biceps		0.43	0.45	0.50	0.30	n.s.	0.30	0.33	0.19
Triceps			0.42	0.51	0.37	n.s.	0.47	0.46	0.35
Subscapular				0.61	0.46	0.23	0.52	0.52	0.27
Suprailiac					0.46	0.25	0.65	0.67	0.38
Sum 4 SFT					0.51	0.21†	0.62†	0.64	0.37
12 months	Biceps	Triceps	Sub-scapular	Supra-iliac	BMI	A pp	Asag sc	Aax sc	R sc/pp
PI	0.41	0.43	0.54	0.43	0.92	0.20	0.51	0.52	0.45
Armcircumf.	0.42	0.51	0.49	0.40	0.65	0.22	0.42	0.39	0.29
Biceps		0.41	0.48	0.56	0.42	0.23	0.47	0.46	0.35
Triceps			0.52	0.42	0.51	0.24	0.44	0.43	0.32
Subscapular				0.63	0.60	0.42	0.70	0.68	0.47
Suprailiac					0.47	0.32	0.68	0.70	0.53
Sum 4 SFT					0.64	0.39†	0.71†	0.71	0.51
Waist					0.64	0.26	0.51	0.49	0.25

† shown in **Figure 22**; n=152 at 6 weeks pp, n=155 at 4 months pp, n=153 at 12 months pp

Results

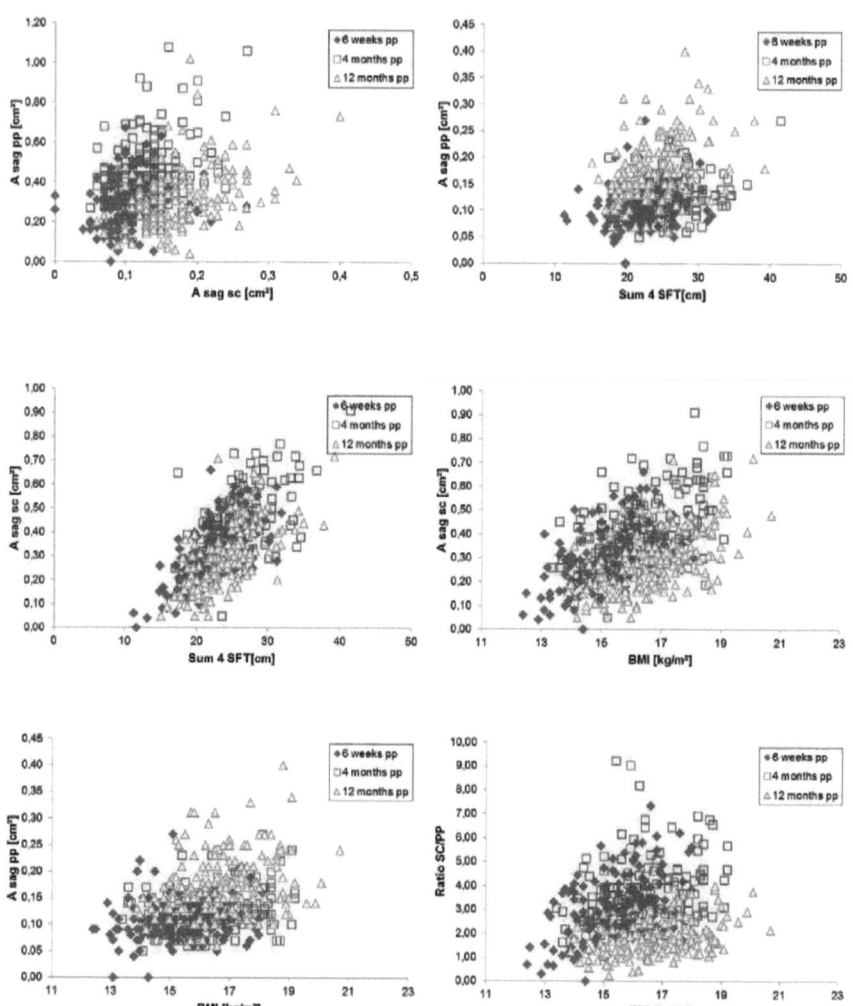

Figure 22: Relationship of the different fat measures among each other stratified by the time point of investigation: diamond (blue)= 6 weeks pp; quadrangle (red) 4 months pp; triangle (red) = 12 months pp; the correlation coefficients are shown in Table 26, 27 and 28.

5 DISCUSSION

5.1 Clinical results (Paper I)

To our knowledge, the INFAT study is the first prospective RCT to test the hypothesis that a reduction of the n-6/n-3 LCPUFAs ratio in the maternal diet may cause less expansive adipose tissue growth in infants. The analyses of this study did not provide evidence that the intervention with fish-oil capsules (1020 mg DHA + 180 mg EPA/d) combined with an AA balanced diet during pregnancy and lactation affected adipose tissue growth and distribution in offspring during the first year of life as shown by 2 methods of body fat assessment (ie, SFT measurement and ultrasonography). The only significant intervention outcome observed was a prolonged gestation by almost 5 d within the term range (37th and 42nd wk of gestation) in the intervention group, together with increased offspring birth weight and growth indexes. The latter differences were likely due to prolonged gestation, and they disappeared within the first year of life.

The hypothesis tested was based on several observations [eg. early in vitro and in vivo studies indicated that n-6 PUFAs, in particular AA, promote adipogenesis (Massiera et al. 2003; Gaillard et al. 1989), whereas n-3 fatty acids rather counteract this process (Ailhaud and Guesnet 2004)]. In addition, animal studies have shown that the n-6/n-3 PUFA ratio is critical for adipose tissue growth (Azain 2004), and human observational studies pointed to a link between the fatty acid composition of breast milk and risk of childhood obesity (Ailhaud et al. 2006).

In view of the current concept of developmental origins of health and diseases (Gluckman and Hanson 2008) and adipogenesis in humans, the novelty and strengths of our RCT are that the intervention started close to the first appearance of adipocytes in the human fetus that occurred between weeks 14 and 16 of gestation (Poissonnet et al. 1983) and lasted until the end of lactation, and early adipose tissue growth and distribution were examined in a precise and longitudinal manner by several complementary methods. Overall, the study concept was designed to contribute to novel insights into the development of early preventive strategies against childhood obesity.

As regards the body fat analysis, SFT measurement is a validated and reproducible method to determine subcutaneous fat in neonates and young infants (Schmelzle and Fusch 2002; Koo et al. 2004) and recently, ultrasonography has been evaluated in infants aged 1–2 y (Holzhauer et al. 2009).

To our knowledge, the INFAT study is the first study to apply ultrasonography for subcutaneous and preperitoneal fat–layer measurements in the first year of life, which, thereby, complemented our anthropometric data set. The statistical and regression analyses of our data showed that the initially observed effect of the intervention on offspring growth (ie. weight, length, head circumference, and adipose tissue growth and distribution) was due to the prolonged gestation, but was not a direct effect of the intervention. In line with our results, a recent Cochrane review (Delgado-Noguera et al. 2010) similarly concluded that maternal n-3 LCPUFAs supplementation during pregnancy and lactation has no impact on child weight in the short, medium, or long term.

Most importantly, compared with other perinatal n-3 LCPUFAs–supplementation trials, this study was the first prospective RCT to be originally designed to investigate the effect of the n-6/n-3 LCPUFAs ratio in the diet of pregnant women and breastfeeding mothers specifically on adipose tissue growth in their offspring as the primary outcome. Several n-3 LCPUFAs–supplementation trials performed in the gestation and/or

Discussion

lactation period have primarily focused on other developmental outcomes of the children [eg. neurodevelopment (Helland et al. 2003; Dunstan et al. 2008; Jensen et al. 2005; Lauritzen et al. 2005b), visual acuity (Jensen et al. 2005; Lauritzen et al. 2004), or allergic disease (Anandan et al. 2009)], and a few of the trials merely reported on weight and length or BMI (Helland et al. 2001; Helland et al. 2008; Lauritzen et al. 2005a; Bergmann et al. 2007; Bergmann et al. 2012, Escolano-Margarit et al. 2011), but not on adipose tissue growth and distribution as recently reviewed by Muhlhausler et al (Muhlhausler et al. 2010).

To date, 5 retrospective analyses of 4 RCTs addressed the potential role of perinatal n-3 LCPUFAs supplementation on BMI in infancy and childhood and came to inconclusive results (Helland et al. 2008; Lauritzen et al. 2005a; Bergmann et al. 2007; Bergmann et al. 2012; Escolano-Margarit et al. 2011; Asserhoj et al. 2009). In this context, there are major differences between our RCT and the previously mentioned studies. Apart from the primary outcome variable, there were considerable differences in the mode and timing of interventions, dosing of DHA (which range from 200 to 1180 mg/d), compliance, and other methodologic aspects. In all trials, children were older (21 and 30 mo and 3, 4, 6, and 7 y) at BMI assessment than the children in our study, and only one of the studies reported SFT data at the end of a maternal LCPUFAs supplementation that lasted for the first 4 mo of lactation (Lauritzen et al. 2005a).

Adipose tissue growth during early life is considered to be a critical determinant of risk of becoming obese later in life because infants who are at the highes end at birth of the distribution for weight or BMI or who grow rapidly during the first 2 y of life seem to be at increased risk of subsequent obesity (Baird et al. 2005). In a recent study, BMI and body weight attained at 1 y of life were shown to have predictive power for the development and persistence of overweight during childhood (Peneau et al. 2011). Furthermore, cellular studies on human body fat suggested that it expands rapidly during the first year of life predominantly by increasing the adipocyte size that subsequently decreases for 1 or 2 y and remains stable for several years (Hager et al. 1977; Knittle et al. 1979). These observations appear to be in accordance with the recent report by Spalding et al (Spalding et al. 2008) that suggested that the fat cell number is fixed early in life.

The most interesting finding of this RCT was the prolonged gestation by almost 5 d in the intervention group together with a higher birth weight. This finding was in agreement with epidemiologic studies (Olsen et al. 1986) and 2 meta-analyses (Makrides et al. 2006; Szajewska et al. 2006) that suggested that marine oils and n-3 LCPUFAs preparations promote a higher birth weight because of prolonged gestation. The biological cause of this effect can be explained by the interference of n-3 LCPUFAs supplementation with uterine prostaglandin production, possibly by inhibiting the production of AA metabolites, primarily prostaglandin E2 and prostaglandin F2a, involved in the initiation of spontaneous labor (Olsen et al. 1986; Makrides et al. 2006).

Our study, which was designed as a proof-of-concept trial, had some additional strengths. There was a well-defined intervention characterized by a high degree of compliance of women with fish-oil capsule intake combined with a concurrent AA-balanced diet during pregnancy and lactation that could be monitored by biomarkers, a low dropout-rate of 18% at the last appointment at 12 mo, and the study population was rather homogenous and able to implement the dietary instructions in their daily lives. Furthermore, the prevalence of breastfeeding was high in both groups.

Limitations of the study were the small sample size, the short observation period to date, and the open-label design of the study. We acknowledge that participants and investigators who performed anthropometric measurements were not blinded to the treatment, and therefore, we could not exclude a potential bias that may have complicated the interpretation of findings. In addition, both the SFT and ultrasound measurements used did not offer a direct measurement of body fat. Furthermore, the known variability in adults regarding the response to this kind of intervention may also have weakened our results, although the major effect was achieved by the supplementation of preformed n-3 LCPUFAs, which may not be affected by individual variability concerning, eg. the FADS genotype. Although maternal prepregnancy weight status and gestational weight gain have been associated with offspring fat mass (Nelson et al. 2010), it is rather unlikely that these variables affected the study outcome because their distribution was balanced between the groups who were randomly assigned. Because our collective was relatively lean (mean prepregnancy BMI ~ 22), our results may not be generalizable to more overweight or obese populations.

In conclusion, our results suggest that the combination of an increased maternal n-3 LCPUFAs exposure and a reduced AA dietary intake during the perinatal period does not affect offspring adipose tissue growth within the first year of life. These data argue against the hypothesis that lowering the n-6/n-3 LCPUFAs ratio may limit adipose tissue growth early in life. However, it cannot be ruled out that the effect of the intervention manifests later in infancy. For this reason, we are running a additional follow-up of the infants to the age of 5 y. The follow-up program also includes regular assessment of diet and physical activity of

5.2 Maternal and cord blood fatty acid profile in relation to infant body composition (Paper II)

In the present study, maternal supplementation with 1200 mg n-3 LCPUFAs/day and a concomitant AA-balanced diet starting from the 15th week of gestation until the 4 months pp, resulted in elevated maternal and cord blood PLs and RBCs concentrations of DHA and EPA and reduced levels of AA in maternal and cord blood lipids, causing a pronounced decrease of the n-6/n-3 LCPUFAs ratio in maternal and cord blood plasma PLs and RBCs.

Since it has been demonstrated that a high-dose maternal n-3 LCPUFAs supplementation is a feasible way to enhance the maternal and neonatal DHA status (van Houwelingen et al. 1995; Connor et al. 1996; Helland et al. 2001) our results are in accordance with such findings. In the entire study population, most LCPUFAs were highly correlated between the neonatal and the maternal (32nd wk) plasma PLs and RBCs fatty acid profile, thus, our data confirm the results of studies in non-supplemented mother-infant pairs (Al et al. 1995; Berghaus et al. 2000; Elias and Innis 2001; Rump et al. 2001), as well as findings in supplemented women (van Houwelingen et al. 1995; Connor et al. 1996; Helland et al. 2001; Krauss-Etschmann et al. 2007).

In some of the previous RCTs in pregnancy reduced levels of maternal/fetal plasma and RBCs n-6 LCPUFAs were reported after n-3 LCPUFAs supplementation (van Houwelingen et al. 1995; Helland et al. 2001; Dunstan et al. 2004; Innis and Friesen 2008), although the reduction was not significant in all studies (Velzing-Aarts et al. 2001; Malcolm 2003; Krauss-Etschmann et al. 2007). It was suggested, that high intakes of EPA plus DHA in the diet, such as from fish oils, might allow for the partial replacement (reduction) of AA in cells and tissues.

In the INFAT-study, we also observed reduced levels of AA in both the maternal and neonatal lipid pools. However, as AA intake at 32nd week of pregnancy was also moderately reduced in the diet of the intervention group (Hauner et al. 2012), we cannot distinguish whether the decrease in blood AA contents was mainly driven by n-3 supplementation or whether the concomitant reduction in dietary AA intake adds further on the AA lowering effects in blood lipids.

The main aim of this analysis was to study the relationship between the n-3 LCPUFAs profile and clinical outcomes, such as pregnancy duration, infant growth and body composition. We found a strong and significant positive association between maternal RBCs DHA, EPA and n-3 LCPUFAs profile and pregnancy duration. This is in line with a Danish study, showing positive effects of n-3 supplementation on gestational length (Olsen et al. 1992). A study performed by Helland (Helland et al. 2001) found higher gestational length in neonates with high plasma PLs DHA. The opposite phenomenon, a negative association, was seen, when maternal RBCs AA and n-6 LCPUFAs contents in late pregnancy were related to gestational age in the present study. This might be explained by the reciprocal effects of n-3 and n-6 LCPUFAs.

Both n-3 LCPUFAs and n-6 LCPUFAs are claimed as indispensable for infant growth and development, yet there is insufficient scientific evidence from existing RCTs to decide whether the individual LCPUFAs profile of either mother or neonate is related to offspring growth (Delgado-Noguera et al. 2010). Most evidence for possible growth-promoting effects of LCPUFAs to date is provided by cohort studies, where birth weight of term infants appeared to be positively associated with maternal n-3 LCPUFAs concentrations, especially DHA, in early pregnancy (van Eijsden et al. 2008; Dirix et al. 2009). However, negative associations between DHA in umbilical cord plasma PLs and neonatal birth weight also have been reported (Rump et al. 2001). The relationship of cord blood/maternal plasma PLs AA contents in pregnancy and at delivery with birth weight was mainly found to be negative (Rump et al. 2001; van Eijsden et al. 2008; Dirix et al. 2009) or rather neutral (Elias and Innis 2001).

Evidence from RCTs is restricted to maternal n-3 LCPUFAs intake and, although positive associations between maternal n-3 LCPUFAs profile and weight dimensions at birth have also been reported, these are commonly interpreted as the consequence of prolonged gestation rather than a direct effect on fetal growth (Makrides et al. 2006; Szajewska et al. 2006). The results of the INFAT-study suggest that maternal RBCs DHA, EPA, total n-3 LCPUFAs, AA, and total n-6 LCPUFAs in the last trimester serve as important fetal growth factors, since these maternal LCPUFAs were found to be significantly positively related to infant weight, length and lean body mass at birth. Of note, this relationship was still apparent after adjustment for cofactors such as pregnancy duration, parity and sex, known to be relevant determinants of fetal growth (Catalano et al. 1995), indicating a direct effect on these fatty acids on growth dimensions. For RBCs DHA, EPA and total n-3 LCPUFAs the observed association with weight and lean body mass at birth was no longer detectable at later stages of infant growth up to the first year of life, suggesting that these fatty acids indeed promote prenatal growth, but do not have an impact on postnatal growth.

On the contrary, maternal RBCs AA and n-6 LCPUFAs were significantly negatively correlated with BMI and Ponderal Index at 1 year of life within the present study. Interestingly, this relationship was still evident after correction for relevant confounders, known to influence perinatal growth (Catalano et al. 1995) and fatty acid profile (van Houwelingen et al. 1995; Helland et al. 2001; Dunstan et al. 2007; van Houwelingen et al. 1999), such as pregnancy duration, sex, parity, growth dimensions achieved at birth and breastfeeding.

This observation might indicate that maternal RBCs n-6 LCPUFAs not only serve as prenatal, but also as a determinant of postnatal overall growth within the first year of life. This surprising finding is hard to explain. However, the observed effects on infant growth, regardless of potential mechanisms (Lapillonne et al. 2003), does not appear to be clinically relevant, because infant weight, length and BMI of the supplemented group was comparable to growth in the control group (Hauner et al. 2012).

Of note, we found a significant negative relationship between umbilical cord blood RBCs concentrations of DHA, EPA and n-3 LCPUFAs with parameters of infant fat mass at birth and 6 weeks pp, but, this association was not detectable at later stages up to age 1y. This result seems in line with the results of Helland et al. observing no significant correlations between cord blood plasma PLs DHA and the ratio of n-6/n-3 fatty acids and children's BMI at 7 years of age (Helland et al. 2008).

Recently, a large US cohort study reported that higher n-3 LCPUFAs concentrations in the maternal diet and in umbilical cord blood plasma PLs are associated with a lower obesity rate in children at 3 years of age, measured by the sum of two skinfold thicknesses (triceps + subscapular), odds of obesity (BMI ≥ 95th percentile compared to BMI < 85th Percentile) and infant leptin, a biomarker directly correlated with obesity (Donahue et al. 2011). These contradictory findings are hard to reconcile, but there is certainly a need for additional studies to address this important issue.

Discussion

The INFAT-study is the first randomized controlled trial to explore in detail the association between individual maternal and fetal LCPUFAs concentrations and infant body fat mass up to the first year of life assessed by skinfold thickness measurements and abdominal ultrasonography.

Maternal RBCs DHA and n-3 LCPUFAs at 32nd week of gestation were significantly positively related with newborn length and lean body mass (g) at birth (estimated by SFT measurements) even when corrected for gestational age, parity, sex and group. We interpret this result more as a growth-promoting, rather than an adipogenic effect of these maternal fatty acids, since particularly lean body mass was positively associated to a greater extent.

This interpretation is further supported by the fact that neither the individual maternal LCPUFAs (DHA, EPA, AA), their sums (n-3 LCPUFAs, n-6 LCPUFAs) or their ratios (AA/DHA, n-6/n-3 LCPUFAs ratio) during late pregnancy were significantly associated with offspring body fat mass as assessed by longitudinal skinfold thickness measurements and abdominal ultrasonography from birth throughout the first year of life. Interestingly, we saw some negative associations between neonatal RBCs EPA, DHA and total n-3 LCPUFAs with single parameters of fat mass (e.g. percentage body fat, subscapular SFT), but not with lean body mass at birth, indicating that circulating LCPUFAs in umbilical cord blood might play some role for adipose tissue growth in the newborns. However, if at all, this effect seems to be confined to the phase around birth, as neither neonatal RBCs DHA, EPA, AA, n-3 LCPUFAs, n-6 LCPUFAs nor the n-6/n-3 LCPUFAs or AA/DHA ratio were significantly correlated with the individual skinfold thicknesses, the sum of the four skinfolds or parameters of fat mass at later stages up to 1 y pp

These findings once more highlight the importance of adequate methods to assess body composition development in early life. Obviously, BMI data alone do not provide sufficient information on body composition and, therefore, should be interpreted with caution. Especially in early infancy, skinfold thickness measurements and sonographic assessment of subcutaneous fat tissues may provide a better assessment of body fat mass and, more indirectly, of lean body mass. BMI data do not distinguish between these two major components of body mass and may promote misinterpretation with regard to the relationship between fatty acids and body composition. Nevertheless, sonographic assessment of body composition might have limited precision in 1 year olds due to the relatively thin fat layers and frequent restlessness of infants (Holzhauer et al. 2009).

Taken together, as already indicated by the analysis of the fatty acid intake data and adipose tissue development (Hauner et al. 2012), this detailed measurements of the fatty acids profile in maternal blood - as well as in umbilical cord blood - do not support the concept that maternal n-3 LCPUFAs exert an anti-adipogenic action, therefore, contradicts previous findings in animal studies (Ailhaud and Guesnet 2004) and available human data with and without such detailed measurements (Donahue et al. 2011; Bergmann et al. 2007, Bergmann et al. 2012). However, to definitely clarify the role of the n-3 LCPUFAs profile and the n-3/n-6 fatty acid balance on infant body composition more long-term studies with appropriate methods to assess adipose tissue development and body composition are necessary.

Supplementation with 1200 mg n-3 LCPUFAs per day and concomitant reduction of AA intake from 15th week of gestation until 4 months postpartum resulted in substantial and expected changes of the fatty acid profile, particularly in a decrease of the ratio of n-6 to n-3 LCPUFAs in maternal and cord blood PLs and RBCs. Maternal DHA, AA and EPA were found to be associated with somatic offspring growth independent of the effects on pregnancy duration. The results also suggest that a reduced maternal n-6/n-3 fatty acid ratio is not associated with adipose tissue expansion during the early postnatal period up to 1 y of age. Further studies with appropriate methods to assess infant body composition in a prospective manner are necessary to further clarify the role of dietary LCPUFAs on long-term infant body composition.

5.3 Breast milk fatty acid profile in relation to infant body composition (Paper III)

The purpose of the present study was to investigate the independent relationship between n-6 vs. n-3 LCPUFAs profile in human breast milk and infant body composition. We hypothesized that proportions of LCPUFAs in breast milk as continuous measures, irrespective of group allocation, are associated with measures of infant growth and body composition within the first year of life.

The underlying association analyses yielded novel results on the differential effects of breast milk fatty acids from the n-3 versus the n-6 fatty acid family on infant fat mass and indices of growth. The central observation was that breast milk n-3 LCPUFAs at 6 wk pp were positively associated with parameters of body fat in the offspring arguing against the hypothesis that a high intake of n-3 LCPUFAs may protect from obesity.

The specific dietary intervention of the INFAT-study was successful, as evidenced by higher n-3 LCPUFAs proportions in breast milk from 6th wk through 4 months pp. Daily supplementation with 1200 mg LCPUFAs (1020mg DHA + 180mg EPA) and a concomitant moderate reduction in maternal AA intake resulted in a significant 5-fold increase in DHA and a 2-fold increase in EPA content in breast milk, without affecting AA concentration. Thus, the specific dietary intervention led to a pronounced decrease in the breast milk n-6/n-3 LCPUFAs ratio up to 4 months pp, which was also clearly reflected by the fatty acid profile in of infant RBCs at the end of the dietary intervention.

An increased secretion of EPA and DHA into human breast milk upon supplementation with fish oil is in agreement with previous observations from n-3 LCPUFAs supplementation RCTs during lactation (Fidler et al. 2000; Helland et al. 2001; Jensen et al. 2005; Lauritzen et al. 2004).

Breast milk AA turned out to be non-responsive to maternal diet, but tightly controlled in the present study. This finding is consistent with previous reports from RCTs (Fidler et al. 2000; Jensen et al. 2005; Lauritzen et al. 2004; Dunstan et al. 2007), describing that n-3 LCPUFAs supplementation during pregnancy and lactation does not decrease the proportions of AA in mature breast milk.

Indeed, breast milk AA is relatively uniform across populations on a worldwide basis (~ 0.24-1.0% of fatty acids) (Brenna et al. 2007), suggesting a physiological and critical role of AA for infant growth and development. Moreover, even the concomitant moderate reduction in dietary AA intake during pregnancy in the present study (Hauner et al. 2012) did not affect breast milk AA content (Breast milk AA at 6 weeks pp: 0.43 ± 0.08 (n=76); in both groups).

The fact that we also did not observe any considerable correlation between maternal RBC and breast milk AA levels gives further support to the suggestion that breast milk AA appears to be under strict physiological control. There is also evidence that the slowly turning-over maternal AA body pool is the major source of milk AA (Del et al. 2001), although this association may be modified by the consumption of AA supplements by lactating mothers (in addition to extra n-3 LCPUFAs), which has been demonstrated to dose dependently increase AA concentrations in breast milk lipids (Weseler et al. 2008).

While the biological variation of breast milk AA is rather low, those of breast milk EPA and DHA content constitute the highest of all fatty acids (Smit et al. 2002; Yuhas et al. 2006), and breast milk concentrations are closely linked to maternal dietary EPA and DHA intake (Makrides et al. 1996).

Little is currently known concerning the role of circulating LCPUFAs in breast milk for adipose tissue growth in the offspring and data from RCT are scarce.

In a Danish trial, mothers with low habitual n-3 fatty acid intake were randomized to receive either fish oil (supplying 0.62 g EPA and 0.79 g DHA per day) or olive oil from 0-4 month of lactation, and the relationship between infant body composition measured by two-sided skinfold thickness investigations and maternal RBC DHA as a biochemical measure of compliance was investigated (Lauritzen et al. 2005a).

The maternal fish oil supplementation during lactation led to an increased BMI and waist circumference at 2.5 years of age. Also, in a subgroup of 60 infants, BMI, waist circumference, triceps SFT and percentage body fat at 2.5 y of age were positively associated with the DHA content of maternal RBCs at the end of the intervention period in adjusted models. Of note, also DHA content in a sample of breast milk taken at 4 months pp was significantly associated with BMI and waist circumference at 2.5y, respectively, but no associations with the sum of triceps + subscapular skinfold thickness was found (Lauritzen et al. 2005a). In the long-term follow up of the children at 7 years of age however, none of the growth or body composition variables were correlated with maternal RBC DHA (Asserhoj et al. 2009).

The Danish study is the only postnatal n-3 LCPUFAs supplementation trial to date performing SFT measurements to determine percentage body fat and thus being able to discriminate between infant fat and lean body mass. However, the trial suffered from a large drop-out rate in the

2.5 y follow-up and exclusively addressed the issue of body composition in post-hoc analyses.

In a trial from Norway investigating women randomized either to cod liver oil or corn oil from 18 wk of pregnancy until 3 months of lactation, Helland et al. found no correlation between the content of n-6 long-chain PUFAs (LA, AA) in breast milk and BMI at the age of 7 years. In contrast, they observed that the content of ALA in breast milk collected at 4 weeks and 3 months after birth was positively correlated with later BMI (Helland et al. 2008).

In our study, we found positive associations between early but not late breast milk LCPUFAs from the 3-series on different measures of infant fat mass across all time-points: DHA, EPA and total n-3 LCPUFAs in early breast milk were consistently and positively associated with the sum of 4 SF at 1 year of age, and for DHA also at 4 months pp. Furthermore, the n-3 fatty acids in breast milk were positively associated with some individual skinfolds at the different time points over the 1st y of life. Late breast milk proportions of DHA, EPA and n-3 LCPUFAs were significantly negatively associated with length 1 y pp, and significantly positively associated with growth indices.

This suggests that, contrary to our original hypothesis, an increased supply of n-3 fatty acids during critical periods of adipose tissue development in the newborn via breast milk stimulates fat accumulation in early postnatal life. This unexpected finding further supports our previous null findings when we compared adipose tissue growth between the intervention and the control group (Hauner et al. 2012).

This finding is also in contrast with former animal data linking an increased n-3 LCPUFAs supply with reduced fat cell differentiation and accumulation in adult rodents and in vitro studies (Massiera et al. 2003;

Oosting et al. 2010) and in offspring of mothers fed with a diet high in n-3 fatty acids during the pregnancy/lactation period (Baird et al. 2005).

Another interesting finding of the present study was that, early breast milk n-6 LCPUFAs including AA showed consistent negative associations with infant body weight, growth parameters, such as BMI and Ponderal Index, as well as with lean body mass (g) up to 4 months postpartum, but not at 1 y of age. Early breast milk n-6 LCPUFAs were also significantly negatively related to individual SFT (e.g. triceps, suprailiac SFT), the sum 4 SFT and percentage body up to 6 weeks pp.

This suggests that early breast milk fatty acids from the n-6 fatty acid family serve as important regulating factors for growth in early postnatal life, and particularly of growth of fat and lean body mass.

We, therefore, speculate that from an evolutionary perspective it might be plausible that AA secretion in breast milk is highly regulated to ensure the growth-regulating effects of breast milk AA on body weight, and particularly lean body mass, in the breastfed infant. Due to the low variability of AA-contents in breast-milk, the ingested volume as defined by the daily amount of milk intake by the breast-fed infant might play a critical role in growth-regulatory effects of AA, too. We therefore encourage further studies to look into such quantitative aspects, as well.

In contrast, *early* breast milk fatty acids from the n-3 fatty acid family, thus DHA, EPA, or total n-3 LCPUFAs, were not associated with growth indices or lean body mass up to the first year of life, suggesting different functional roles of LCPUFAs from the n-6 vs. n-3 fatty acid series in postnatal growth. Of note, the AA/DHA and the total n-3/n-6 LCPUFAs ratio were significantly negatively correlated with BMI at 6 weeks pp, but not associated with any of the other outcomes under study up to 1 y pp.

Our latter finding is supported by a very recent analysis of the Copenhagen Prospective Study on Asthma and Childhood, a cohort study primarily designed to assess children born to atopic mothers. Pedersen et al. (2012) observed no associations between breast-milk n-6/n-3 polyunsaturated fatty acid ratio at ~3 weeks postpartum and body composition assessed by dual energy X-ray absorptiometry between the age of 2-7 y. Interestingly, the Danish study found an inverse relationship between breast-milk DHA and parameters of child growth, observed by changes in the timing of adiposity rebound, BMI from 2-7y, and body fat mass, suggesting that high DHA supply to the breastfed infant might delay the age at adiposity rebound. These results have to be confirmed in long-term interventional trails in a non-atopic population.

A strength of the INFAT-study is that the breast milk samples were collected at two different time points over the breastfeeding period (6 weeks, 4 months). This enabled us to investigate the association of both the early and late breast milk LCPUFAs profile with infant growth and body fat mass development at different postnatal ages. Thereby, we unraveled marked differences in the regulatory function of breast milk LCPUFAs in early and later postnatal nutrition, with early breast milk n-3 LCPUFAs being the more important drivers of postnatal fat mass growth.

It is rather unlikely that LCPUFAs from another source than breast milk have distorted the associations between the fatty acid composition of the breast milk and infant fat mass. As 95 % of the women in both groups in the present study decided to breastfeed their infants and the duration of exclusive breastfeeding was on average 20 wk, the proportion of fatty acids present in breast milk is expected to reflect the amount of LCPUFAs ingested by the infants.

We cannot exclude that genetic variants have modified the association between fish oil intake and DHA proportions in human milk. Recently a Dutch study provided evidence that a high fish (or fish oil) intake in women homozygous for the minor allele for a certain FADS1/2 variant was able to compensate for their lower DHA proportions in plasma phospholipids, but not in their milk compared with carriers of the major allele (Molto-Puigmarti et al. 2010). However, such gene-diet interactions in LCPUFAs metabolism remain to be confirmed in larger studies.

As recently suggested in a narrative review by Decsi and Boehm (in press) including own research data, also, trans isomeric fatty acids in human breast mik may have disturbed the availability of LCPUFAs in the perinatal period: in a sizeable group of German mothers donating breast milk samples at 6th week and 6 months of lactation, the authors found, that the 18-carbon trans fatty acid was significantly inversely correlated with DHA and AA proportions in breast milk. Analysis of the trans fatty acid data is currently underway to address this issue within the INFAT study as well.

Our study is limited by providing data on body composition only over a short period in infancy and childhood, respectively, and thus does not allow final conclusions on long-term body weight and in particular body fat development. Results from the long-term follow-up of the participants and data from other on-going RCTs have to be awaited before drawing definite conclusions on the long-term consequences of an increased perinatal n-3 LCPUFAs intake or reduced n-6/n-3 LCPUFAs ratio on infant body composition.

The results of our study suggest that breast milk n-3 LCPUFAs at 6 wk pp appear to stimulate fat mass growth over the 1st year of life, whereas AA seems to be involved in the regulation of overall growth especially in the early postpartum period. The fatty acid ratio in breast milk does not seem to be a critical determinant in infant adiposity development. However, results from long-term follow-up investigations are necessary before drawing robust conclusions.

5.4 Sonographic assment of fat mass and fat distribution and its relation to anthropometry and skinfold thickness measurements (Paper IV)

To the best of our knowledge, this is the first study to apply ultrasonography as measurement technique for the investigation of fat distribution in infants aged ≤ 1 year. All previous studies quantified infant fat mass by rather indirect methods, such as length, weight, calculation of BMI, or assessment of skinfold thickness and waist circumference (Bergmann et al. 2007; Bergmann et al. 2012, Owens et al. 1999; Wells and Fewtrell 2006). In this study, ultrasonography was established as a valid and easy-to-perform bed-side method to quantify abdominal subcutaneous and preperitoneal fat tissue in early infancy.

5.4.1 Method and reproducibility

In recent studies, the technique of sonographic assessment of preperitoneal and subcutaneous adipose tissue has been validated in adults and older children (Liu et al. 2003; Soyama et al. 2005; Suzuki et al. 1993). Holzhauer et al. were the first to establish a protocol in infants by investigating 212 1-year and 227 2-year olds, respectively (Holzhauer et al. 2009).

Ultrasonography is a non-invasive, easy to handle and quickly performable technique. Therefore, it is particularly applicable in early childhood and infancy. In the present study, sonographic assessment of adipose tissue was applied in the upper quadrant of the abdomen according to the method of Holzhauer et al. (Holzhauer et al. 2009) with slight modifications. The abdominal area is particularly useful for the exact quantification of adipose tissue mass, because an echo-rich fascia well discriminates the two fat depots of interest (SC, PP). At evaluation, this fascia functions as the ventral, while the liver acts as the dorsal/intra-abdominal border of preperitoneal fat. Thus, a very well differentiation between subcutaneous and preperitoneal fat layers is possible. In caudal direction the discrimination is hardly possible because of the aeriferous intestine. Moreover, the upper abdomen provides suitable anatomical reference structures, such as the sternum for the assessment of the sagittal area or the linea alba, the fissure of connective tissue between the muscle groups of the M. rectus abdominis for measuring the axial area. These reference structures were essential for the optimal standardization of the method.

The reproducibility of our investigation was good to excellent. Precision was calculated by intraclass-correlation coefficients (ICC) and the error of precision EP_{RMS}. The results were in agreement with the intra-observer data of the study of Holzhauer et al. in infants aged 1 and 2 years (Holzhauer et al. 2009).

Difficulties in the quality of the pictures and during the evaluation were caused by several factors. The frequent restlessness in the small participants was problematic as it often resulted in movement artifacts. To calm down the infants a silent, warm tempered atmosphere and the presence of the parents was essential. The investigations required patience in the work with the infants, who were often appeased by non-nutritive sucking of a glucose dilution or their soother, or by a musical clock or other tools. However, in some infants the investigation was only possible while sleeping resulting in prolonged investigation times. The cooperation of the infants improved with increasing age, which was also reflected by an reduction in the error of precision (e.g. EP_{RMS} Asag pp at 6 weeks: 8.8%, 1 y pp: 4.8%; EP_{RMS} Aax sc at 6 weeks: 7.2%, 1 y pp: 2.7%) by age.

Another problem was caused by the increased breathing-intensity of the infants, with frequencies of 25-30/min, compared to the adult population. In previous studies in adolescents or adults (Tamura et al. 2000; Tanaka et al. 2005), the measurements were performed in deemed expiration, however, this procedure is not applicable in such a young pediatric population. To use a standardized breathing-phase anyhow, we used the tool of the cine-loop-function which is often integrated in the newer ultrasound systems. By this specific function, it was possible to save the last 63 images taken and after "de-freezing" all individual images could be displayed. Therefore, it was possible to identify single images taken in maximal expiration. An example for the variation of preperitoneal fat thickness stratified by breathing-intensity is demonstrated in **Figure 23**.

The biggest variance was observed at the preperitoneal caudal (sag, caudal pp) points of measurement. A possible explanation for this might be that the liver possesses a high breathing dislocation, but serves as a reference structure at the same time. Therefore the measurement of preperitoneal fat was much more affected by the breathing-movements than the measurement of the subcutaneous fat layers (**Figure 23**).

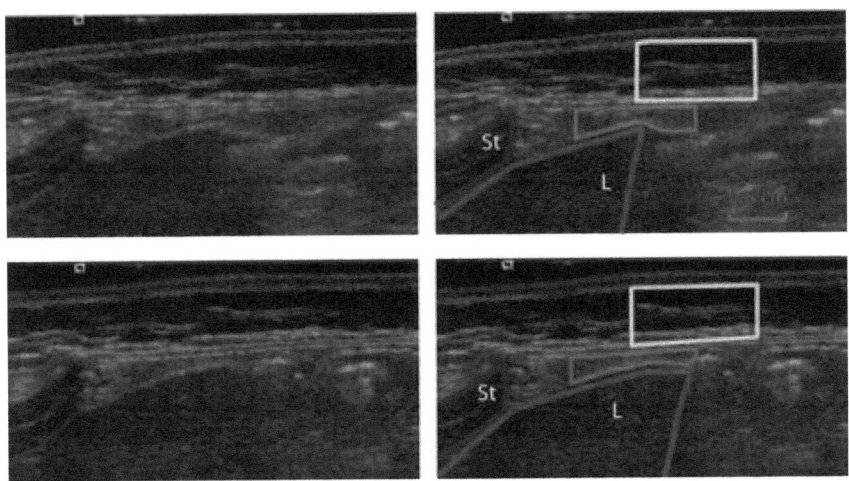

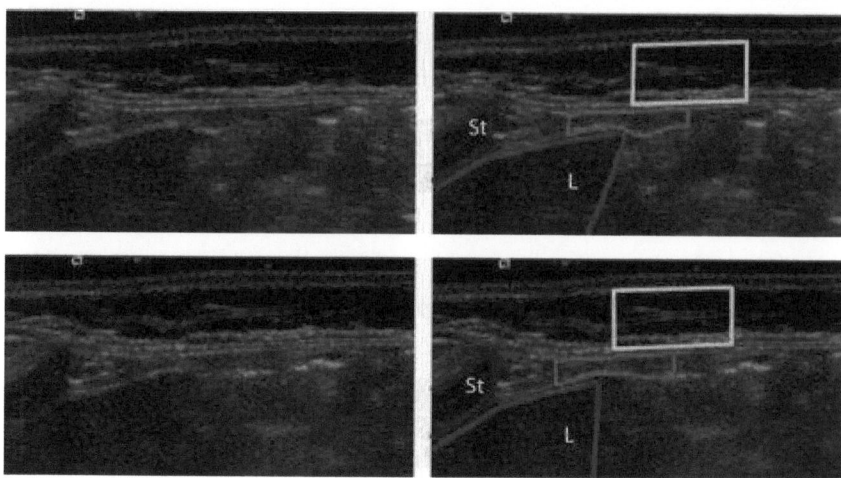

Figure 23: Examples of measuring subcutaneous and preperitoneal fat layers in different breathing phases; the subcutaneous fat layer (yellow) remains unaffected. Preperitoneal fat layer (red) changes depending on the breathing phase. During inspiration (top) the liver shifts (green) towards distal direction (right picture) with the sternum as reference point (blue), with increasing expiration (Figure downwards) the liver is shifted below the sternum Sternum. St: Sternum. L: Liver.

Discussion

In the retrospective evaluation of the ultrasound pictures, some images showed increased echo within the subcutaneous fat layer, which complicated the identification of the reference points and resulted in getting inaccuracy. These within-echo were mainly caused by the structures of connective tissue located within the subcutaneous adipose tissue layers (example **Figure 24**)

For standardization, the within-echo was included in the measurement and the evaluators (E.H., D.M.) agreed to set the reference point as closely to the fascia as possible.

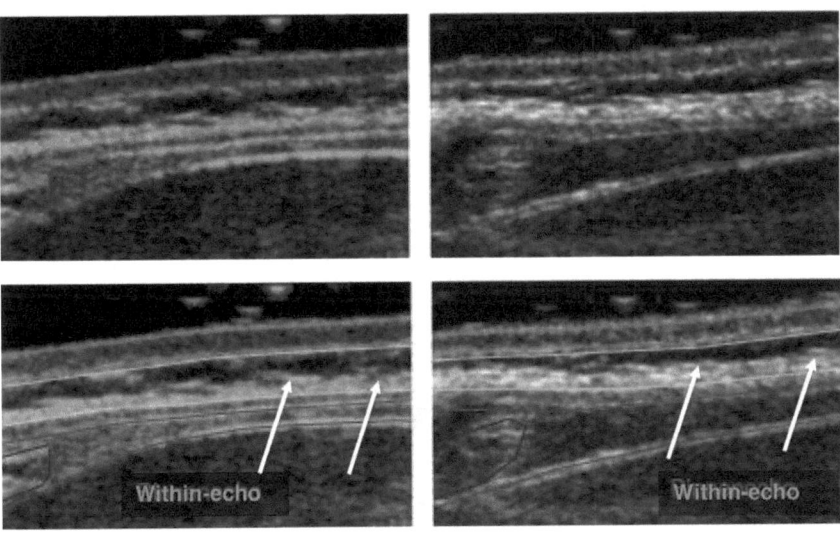

Figure 24: Examples (down with marked labeling) for demonstration of the different within-echo (arrow) within the subcutaneous adipose tissue (yellow areal) and for different echogenecity of preperitoneal fat tissue (red areal) with increasingly higher echogenicity in the left picture. The cutis is labeled orange; the sternum is labeled blue.

Discussion

In summary, an adequate training and operating experience of the observer were essential for successful performance of the investigation. A part of the pictures was evaluated by two different observers (E.H., D.M.) to calculate interobserver variance. The results from interobserver-analyses showed good agreement (Table 23) and were comparable with the findings of the study of Holzhauer et al. The highest comparability was observed in the calculation of the preperitoneal area. We believe, that this is explained by the fact that it is especially this district where the observers had the highest certainty where to set the reference points, because this area of fat tissue generally showed very little within-echo.

Holzhauer et al. (2009) found the best results after calculation of an area with the length of 2 cm and recommended to standardize this technique. However, this evaluation was not reproducible by our measurements; the small size of this area in our age group did not allow for measurement of an area of 2cm length in the preperitoneal fat layer. For better comparability, we therefore recommend the calculation of an area with 1cm length, at least for investigations during the first year of infancy.

To definitively establish ultrasonography for the assessment of fat distribution in early infancy, age-specific validation with other direct methods such as MRI or computer tomography (CT) is needed. Thereby it is especially warranted to investigate or confirm the association between preperitoneal fat assessed by ultrasonography with intra-abdominal fat mass in infancy. Mook-Kanamori et al. (2009) were the first to compare preperitoneal fat with visceral fat in 47 nonobese children (aged 7.9 y) by CT. Moreover, they compared CT measurements with ultrasonographic assessment of abdominal fat distribution in 34 children (aged 9.7 y). Their findings suggest that preperitoneal fat can be used as an approximation of visceral fat for children and that measuring of abdominal fat in children is a valid method for epidemiological and clinical studies, whereas the exact agreement between ultrasonography and CT was limited. Similar analyses in infants aged ≤ 1 y are lacking to date, therefore the question remains open whether preperitoneal fat is a measure of intra-abdominal fat at that age group. To close that gap, a small collective of the infants was scanned by MRI technique in the current study (n=36). Analyses of the fat depots are currently ongoing and performed by cooperation-partners from the Institute of Radiology, Technische Universität München.

5.4.2 Adipose tissue development and sex differences

To the best of our knowledge, this is the first study to provide information on the development of different fat depots by a direct measuring technique within the first year of infancy. Previous data rather relied on indirect methods such as assessment of height, weight, BMI or skinfold thickness measurements (Bergmann et al. 2007; Owens et al. 1999; Wells and Fewtrell 2006). Holzhauer et al. assessed fat distribution and adipose tissue development within the second year of life (Holzhauer et al. 2009). Thereby, they found a rapid increase in the thickness of the preperitoneal fat layer, whereas in contrary the subcutaneous adipose tissue showed no increase. Consequently, this resulted in a shift in the abdominal fat tissue-ratio towards an increase in preperitoneal fat mass. Our study showed that both fat depots, SC and PP fat, were increasing up to 4 months postpartum. These findings are in accordance with the study data from Olhager et al., who investigated adipose tissue development of 46 infants by MRI technique within their first 4 months of life (Olhager et al. 2003). They found an increase in subcutaneous adipose tissue, as well as in non-subcutaneous fat layers within the first 4 months of infancy, with more than 90% of the fat mass being located in the subcutaneous region.

Over the further course of the study, preperitoneal fat thickness significantly increased during the first year of life (App 10.7 mm^2 at 6 weeks pp vs. 13.1 mm^2 at 4 months vs. 17.9 mm^2 at 1y pp), whereas subcutaneous adipose tissue was significantly lower at 12 months of age compared to 4 months pp, and was even lower than 6 weeks pp (Asag sc 30.8 mm^2 vs. 41.5 mm^2 vs. 28.4 mm^2). These observations suggest that there already exist different stages of adipose tissue development within the first year of life. We could show that the shift in abdominal fat distribution, which was previously described by Holzhauer et al. within the second year of life, seems to start much earlier in infancy. Recent studies on adipose tissue growth described an increase of fat mass from 13-16% at birth up to 28% until the first year of life, which was mainly a result from fat deposition in the subcutaneous regions (Fischer-Posovszky 2004). In the beginning of the 20th century, Stratz described different phases in adipose tissue growth, each characterized by specific changes (Stratz 1902), e.g. the first year of life was described as the "first filling period", followed by a reduction of subcutaneous adipose tissue starting within the second year of life. On the contrary, the data of the present study suggest a much earlier start in the decline of subcutaneous and the increase in preperitoneal fat mass. Therefore, further studies of longitudinal design with different assessments over the first year of life are warranted to detect when exactly the shift in the SC/PP ratio towards an increase in preperitoneal fat mass takes place and to identify possible factors which contribute to this process.

The comparison of adipose tissue growth between the sexes assessed by ultrasonography revealed significant differences between girls and boys, e.g. at 6 weeks, 4 months and 12 months pp the subcutaneous fat layer was significantly thicker in females than in males. These findings are in accordance with previous studies reporting a higher relative fat mass and higher subcutaneous fat in girls starting from 1 year of life compared with boys or young men of the same age group (Fox et al. 1993; Geer and Shen 2009; Kuk et al. 2005). Preritoneal fat thickness was not significantly different between boys and girls at any time point investigated (p>0.05). This observation is in contrast to the results of studies reporting higher visceral fat mass in 11-year-old boys (Fox et al. 1993) as well as in adults. Holzhauer et al. (2009) even found higher preperitoneal fat thickness in girls at both, 1 and 2 years of age. These data were confirmed by a British trial including n=170 infants with an average age of 13y (Benfield et al. 2008), where adipose tissue distribution was investigated by MRI technique. These contrary findings compared to our results are hard to explain. Therefore, the results from the follow-up investigations have to be awaited before final conclusions regarding the impact of sex differences in adipose tissue development can be drawn.

5.4.3 Correlations of the different fat measures

In the present study, the comparison of sonograpic parameters with the different anthropometric measures within the first year of life showed a moderate correlation between subcutaneous fat mass and BMI (Aax sc and BMI: $r = 0.60$ or Asag sc and BMI: $r = 0.57$ at 6 wk pp; Table 26), whereas preperitoneal fat was rather found to be weakly correlated to BMI (r = n.s. at 6 wk pp; $r< 0.27$ at 4 months and 12 months pp). These results were independent of age and sex. Thus, the results confirm observations from several studies comparing the different methods of assessment and describing BMI as a predictor for subcutaneous fat mass in different age groups and with different measuring techniques (Brambilla et al. 2006; Holzhauer et al. 2009; Oka et al. 2009). Holzhauer et al. (2009) investigated 1 to 2-y olds by ultrasonography and compared the data with BMI and waist circumference and they found a moderate association between BMI and subcutaneous fat mass. Oka et al. (Oka et al. 2009) compared waist circumference and BMI with visceral and subcutaneous fat mass assessed by CT in adult men and women aged 38-60 y. Brambilla et al. (2006) collected BMI and waist circumference data of 497 children aged 7-16 y and associated them with visceral and subcutaneous fat evaluated by magnetic resonance imaging (MRI) technique. They found waist circumference as predictor for intra-abdominal fat mass and BMI as a predictor for subcutaneous fat mass. These data were confirmed in the present study in infants ≤ 1 y. Preperitonal fat had the highest correlation (r = 0.42) with subscapular SFT at 1y pp, but correlated rather weakly with other anthropometric measures (e.g. BMI r<0.27 up to 1 y pp).

Han et al. investigated 20 women aged 20-51 y by MRI and 71 men and 34 women with CT. Moreover, an anthropometric dataset such as BMI, waist circumference and SFT was collected. Again, and especially with MRI measurements, waist circumference was identified and confirmed as best predictor of intra-abdominal fat mass. Of interest an impact of age was detected, because older people had more intra-abdominal fat mass albeit similar waist circumferences. This observation was confirmed in a recent study by Kuk et al (2005) suggesting an effect of hormones which has to be considered when estimating visceral adipose tissue by waist circumference. To study the possible hormonal influences on adipose tissue growth further studies are required.

In summary, we could show that sonography is a valid method with good reproducibility for the quantification of abdominal subcutaneous and preperitoneal adipose tissue in early infancy ≤ 1y. Especially preperitoneal fat tissue was described as an independent, discretely developing fat depot, which is only detectable by ultrasonography or other directs measurement techniques such as MRI or CT. Further studies investigating the relationship between preperitoneal fat and intra-abdominal adipose tissue in infancy are needed. A comparison of preperitonal fat assessed by ultrasonography and intra-abdominal fat mass quantified by MRI or CT should necessarily be carried out to approve the possible association. We could show, that a shift in the ratio of SC/PP fat already occurs before the completion of the first year of life. A study collecting the anthropometric dataset at closer intervals should be conducted to detect the exact time point of change in fat distribution and to identify possible influencing factors.

6 CONCLUSION AND FURTHER PERSPECTIVES

The INFAT trial is a proof-of-concept study to test the hypothesis that lowering the n-6/n-3 long-chain fatty acid ratio in the diet of pregnant/breastfeeding women may reduce the expansion of adipose tissue growth early in life and may, thereby, represent a completely novel approach for the primary prevention of childhood obesity (Hauner et al. 2009). This research question goes back to G. Ailhaud who was the first to describe the pro-adipogenic effect of arachidonic acid and the counteracting effect of long-chain n-3 PUFAs, first in cell culture models and later in animal experiments (Ailhaud et al. 2006). Similar animal data have been published by other groups (Muhlhausler et al. 2011b; Oosting et al. 2010).

Post-hoc retrospective analyses of human intervention studies using mainly DHA and looking at BMI as secondary endpoint gave conflicting results and had severe limitations (Muhlhausler et al. 2010). Our study is the first to directly address this issue in a prospective RCT in humans and is thus timely in relation to the on-going discussions in the field. It represents more a proof-of-concept study and was performed in a single center with the advantage of highly standardized methods and a well-trained study team. Repeated measurements over time and several state-of-the-art methods to assess infant fat mass (primary endpoint) were used (Hauner et al. 2009).

The results of our study do not verify the original hypothesis because we found no anti-obesity effects of the intervention to reduce the n-6/n-3 fatty acid ratio between the randomized groups (Paper I) (Hauner et al. 2012). Likewise, complementary association analyses in the whole sample revealed no anti-obesity properties of circulating maternal or neonatal n-3 LCPUFAs (or a reduced n-6/n-3 LCPUFAs ratio) (Paper II), supporting our previous null finding in the group comparison. Thus, the results of our study challenge the prevailing hypothesis that high n-3 LCPUFAs levels of pregnant women and lactating mothers decrease adiposity in their offspring. We believe that the study results provide clear and robust data and make an important contribution to clarify this topic which received broad attention in recent years and may be highly relevant for the upcoming issue of fetal programming in man.

It is important to note, that our study and the before mentioned trials only provide data on body composition over a limited period in infancy or childhood, respectively, and do not allow final conclusions on long-term body weight and in particular body fat development. However, given the well-documented persistence of adiposity status between infancy/childhood and the adult age (Baird et al. 2005) and the widely accepted view of early life representing a critical period of adipose tissue development where the number of adipocytes is likely to be set (Spalding et al. 2008), these data might serve as a suitable indicator for subsequent adiposity development at later stages (Hauner et al., in press).

Our study provides comprehensive and novel insights into the physiological functions of LCPUFAs from the n-3 and the n-6 family on infant growth and body composition during critical periods: Circulating maternal DHA and AA contents during late pregnancy were found to be associated with somatic offspring growth at birth and pregnancy duration revealing an important role of these fatty acids during the intrauterine period (Paper II). Postnatal n-3 LCPUFAs supply via breast milk at 6 weeks pp was positively associated with parameters of body fat in the offspring through the 1st y of life arguing against the hypothesis that a high intake of n-3 LCPUFAs may protect from obesity. Interestingly, breast milk n-6 LCPUFAs were significantly associated with offspring growth, thereby unraveling different regulatory properties of the breast milk fatty acids from the n-6 and n-3 family on infant growth and body composition in the postnatal phase (Paper III).

Our study is not the first trial which did not show beneficial effects of n-3 LCPUFAs on health outcomes in the randomized participants. Although n-3 LCPUFAs are widely marketed by the industry as healthy and beneficial for mother and infant when consumed during pregnancy and also many experts recommend fish oil intake during pregnancy, evidence from RCTs does not demonstrate a clear and consistent benefit of n-3 LCPUFAs supplementation during pregnancy and/or lactation on term infants growth, neurodevelopment and visual acuity (Dziechciarz et al. 2010; Campoy et al. 2012). Also no preventive effects on adverse pregnancy outcomes such as preterm birth (Makrides et al. 2006; Larqué et al. 2012), gestational diabetes (GDM) (Zhou et al. 2012) and preeclampsia (Makrides et al. 2006; Zhou et al. 2012) or maternal depressive symptoms could be established (Jans et al. 2010) to date, although null-findings of the latter should be interpreted with caution due to methodological limitations in this research area. Although one may have expected positive effects of increased fish oil uptake during pregnancy for offspring cardiovascular system, no reduction in adolescent blood pressure or heart rate at 19-y of age could be detected in a recent follow-up of a large RCT (Rytter et al. 2012). In contrast, n-3 LCPUFAs supplementation during pregnancy might be a promising strategy for the reduction of allergic biomarkers in infancy (Larqué et al. 2012).

It is tempting to speculate that the genetic heterogeneity in fatty acid metabolism (eg polymorphisms in FADS1/2) may be one of the reasons (besides differences in study design and/or quality) for the apparent inconsistent results of several studies that investigated the effects of a perinatal n-3 LCPUFAs supplementation on clinical outcomes. This new important confounder has to be taken into consideration in future RCTs to clarify possible gene-nutrient interactions and to enhance study sensitivity and precision (Campoy et al. 2012).

However, before DHA supplementation in pregnancy becomes widespread, it is important to know not only if there are benefits, but also if any risks exist for either the mother or child and large scale intervention trials are currently underway to address this issue critically (Makrides et al. 2010).

When the idea goes back to the prevention of childhood obesity, multiple perinatal factors, most of them modifiable, have been shown to be associated with subsequent obesity development in the offspring (Hauner et al., in press). Evidence is accumulating that maternal pre-pregnancy BMI and excessive gestational weight gain is positively related to newborn's body fat mass (Hull et al. 2011), but also offspring's body mass index and BMI from infancy trough adulthood (Crozier et al. 2010; Fraser et al. 2010; Schack-Nielsen et al. 2010).

Obesity is common among women of childbearing age. Epidemiological data from the United Kingdom suggested that first trimester maternal obesity has been significantly increasing over time, having more than doubled from 7.6% to 15.6% from 1989-2007 (Heslehurst et al. 2010). Voigt et al. estimated the prevalence of obesity in pregnancy in Germany at about 10–11% (Voigt et al. 2008). Recently, results from the Hyperglycemia and Adverse Pregnancy Outcome (HAPO) Study showed that both maternal obesity and gestational diabetes mellitus are independently associated with adverse pregnancy outcomes, such as birth weight > 90. percentile and the combination of the two factors showed a greater risk of adverse pregnancy outcomes than either obesity or GDM alone (Catalano et al. 2012). As recently shown, gestational weight gain is also a strong predictor for post-partum weight retention (Nehring et al. 2011) and contributes to overweight and obesity in women of childbearing age (Mamun et al. 2010). Lifestyle intervention studies comprising physical activity, nutrition counseling and psychological factors relevant to pregnancy are effective tools for adequate gestational weight gain and reduce the rate of associated co-morbidities (Tanentsapf et al. 2011; Skouteris et al. 2010) and possibly childhood adiposity risk.

To monitor childhood obesity over the life span an accurate assessment of neonatal body composition by adequate methods is essential, but their application will remain a challenge in future studies. A variety of methods can be applied to investigate infant body composition, however, all have several limitations and difficulties, e.g. radiation exposure, high inter- or intra-observer variances, or they introduce errors by the variable hydration of fat-free mass in young infants (reviewed by Ellis 2007). In the present study a new, innovative and easy-to-handle method to assess infant body composition and fat distribution was applied. Ultrasonography was established as a reproducible and valid method to assess infant fat mass ≤ 1 y. The results of our study could show that PP fat is a discretely developing fat depot which increases through the first year of life. We also demonstrated that the shift in SC/PP fat distribution already occurs earlier as previously suggested in literature (Holzhauer et al. 2009). A comparison of preperitonal fat assessed by ultrasonography and intra-abdominal fat mass quantified by MRI or CT should necessarily be carried out to approve possible associations (Paper IV).

In conclusion, the health risks of obesity not only depend on the amount of body fat, but also on the distribution of the fat depots and, thus, the importance to detect body composition changes in the pediatric population is gaining recognition. The combination of anthropometry and new imaging techniques must be promoted as gold-standard methodologies in RCTs of modest sample size (n<100) to objectively detect effects of individual nutrients on infant body composition.

Although our current understanding of the multiple factors and mechanisms which contribute to early childhood obesity is rather limited, it was suggested that the avoidance of excessive gestational weight gain, moderate exercise, and a prudent diet are reasonable recommendations until the results of on-going research studies are available (Catalano et al. 2012). Such perinatal interventions might be more promising strategies to prevent childhood obesity than approaches on individual nutrient level (eg. increased perinatal n-3 LCPUFAs uptake).

7 SUMMARY

Background: The composition of long-chain PUFAs (LCPUFAs) in the maternal diet may affect obesity risk in the offspring. It was suggested, that eicosanoids derived from the n-6 LCPUFAs arachidonic acid (AA) might stimulate the hyperplastic development of adipose tissue, while LCPUFAs derived from the n-3 family seem to counteract this process.

Objective: We hypothesized that a reduction in the n-6 (omega-6)/n-3(omega-3) LCPUFAs ratio in the diet of pregnant women and breastfeeding mothers may prevent expansive adipose tissue growth in their infants during the first year of life.

Design: In an open-label randomized controlled trial, 208 healthy pregnant women were randomly assigned to an intervention (1200 mg n-3 LCPUFAs as a supplement per day and a concomitant reduction in AA intake) or a control diet from the 15th wk of pregnancy to 4 mo of lactation. The primary outcome was infant fat mass estimated by skinfold thickness (SFT) measurements at 4 body sites at 3–5 d, 6 wk, and 4 and 12 mo postpartum (pp). Secondary endpoints included pregnancy outcome, fatty acid profile in maternal blood, cord blood and breast milk, infant growth and the sonographic assessment of abdominal subcutaneous (SC) and preperitoneal (PP) fat. A comparison of the randomized groups was conducted. Maternal, neonatal and breast milk LCPUFAs were related to infant growth and body composition. A cross-validation of methods to assess infant body composition was performed.

Results: Dietary intervention significantly reduced the n-6/n-3 LCPUFAs ratio in maternal plasma phospholipids (PLs) and red blood cells (RBCs), cord blood PLs and RBCs and breast milk lipids. Infants did not differ in the sum of their 4 SFTs at ≤ 1 y of life [intervention: 24.1 ± 4.4 mm (n =

85); control: 24.1 ± 4.1 mm (n = 80); mean difference: 20.0 mm (95% CI: 21.3. 1.3 mm)] or in growth in corrected analyses (main confounder, eg. pregnancy duration). Likewise, longitudinal ultrasonography showed no significant differences in abdominal fat mass or fat distribution. No significant association of maternal or neonatal n-3 LCPUFAs and fat mass assessed by SFT and ultrasonography was found during the 1st y of life.

Maternal RBCs DHA, total n-3 LCPUFAs and total n-6 LCPUFAs at the 32nd week of gestation were significantly positively related with birth weight (p<0.05). Maternal total RBCs n-3 LCPUFAs, AA and total n-6 LCPUFAs were significantly positively associated with length at birth and except for AA also with head circumference at birth (p<0.05). Maternal RBCs AA and total n-6 LCPUFAs were significantly negatively related to BMI and Ponderal Index at 1 y pp. High breast-milk n-3 LCPUFAs content in the early postpartum period was associated with fat mass growth through the 1st year of life, while breast-milk AA and n-6 LCPUFAs content at 6 weeks postpartum was significantly negatively associated with weight, BMI, Ponderal Index and lean body mass (g) at 6 weeks and 4 months postpartum, but not at 1 year postpartum. The shift in abdominal fat distribution (SC/PP ratio) already occurs before 1 y pp and thus earlier as previously reported in literature. Preperitoneal fat is an independent fat depot, as demonstrated by ultrasonography.

Conclusions: Our comparison of the randomized groups suggest that a reduced maternal and neonatal n-6/n-3 fatty acid ratio does not appear to play a role in adipogenesis during the fetal and early postnatal period up to 1 y of age. Nevertheless maternal DHA, total n-3 LCPUFAs, AA and total n-6 LCPUFAs might serve as prenatal growth factors, while n-6 LCPUFAs also seems to regulate postnatal growth. Breast milk n-3 LCPUFAs appear to stimulate fat mass growth over the 1st year of life, whereas AA and n-6 LCPUFAs seem to be involved in the regulation of overall growth especially in the early postpartum period as shown by the pooled analysis. Ultrasonography is a valid method of good reproducibility for the quantification of abdominal subcutaneous and preperitoneal fat mass in infants ≤ 1y of age. Prospective long-term studies using adequate body composition techniques are needed to explore the efficacy of this dietary approach for primary prevention. This trial was registered at clinicaltrials.gov as NCT00362089.

8 ACKNOWLEDGEMENTS

First of all I would like to express my sincere gratitude to Prof. Dr. Hans Hauner, my tutor, for giving me the opportunity to start working in his group in 2008. I am thankful for education, help, encouragement and critical discussion throughout the 4 years of my PhD-studies.

I want to say many thanks to my supervisor, Dr. Ulrike Amann-Gasser, for giving me the professional input I needed, but also for initiating my very personal development.

I want to express my gratitude to my colleague and friend, Stefanie Brunner, for her generous support throughout the last 3 years.

Thank you, Dr. Christiane Vollhardt for introducing me in the daily work of a running RCT. Thank you for perfect interim analyses of the fatty acids data.

I want to thank all my colleagues at the EKFZ, with special thanks to Dr. Bernhard Bader, Eva-Maria Sedlmeier, Dr. Daniela Schmid and Dr. Christina Holzapfel.

This work is a large cooperative project and would not have been possible without the helpful hands of our partners:

I thank Verena Schulte, physician, and Dr. Ellen Heimberg, pediatrician, for performing the ultrasound measurements in the infants. Thank you, Ellen for the great interim analyses of the sonographic dataset.

I want to thank Prof. Dr. Boehm for fruitful discussion and helpful comments with the fatty acids data in busy times of publication. You have been like a second tutor to me.

I really have to thank Dr. Nana Bartke from Danone Research, for co-reading and discussing the lipids part of my papers. Thank you both,

Angelika Green and Michael Möbius, for technical assistance and fatty acid analyses in "epidemic" dimensions.

It is impossible to express in mere words my gratitude to our biostatisticians, Dr. Tibor Schuster and Monika Brüderl, M.Sc. Thank you so much for data analyses.

I also thank Prof. Dr. Rummeny and Dr. Jan Bauer from the Institute of Radiology, for giving us free access to the ultrasonographic system.

I am grateful to the practice-based gynecologists for recruitment support and to midwives of the outpatient departments of obstetrics for their involvement in the trial.

Finally I want to thank all the families and their infants for participating in the INFAT-trial. Special thanks go to my own wonderful family for their generous support.

APPENDIX

APPENDIX 1: Blood coagulation parameters

	group	n	15th wk gest mean ± SD	N	32nd wk gest mean ± SD	n	6th wk pp mean ± SD	n	4th mo pp mean ± SD
Erythrocytes [/pL]	Intervention	103	4.2 ± 0.3	93	3.9 ± 0.3	75	4.5 ± 0.3	63	4.7 ± 0.3
	Control	102	4.2 ± 0.4	94	4.0 ± 0.3	74	4.6 ± 0.4	60	4.8 ± 0.4
Haematocrit [%]	Intervention	103	36.9 ± 2.7	93	34.9 ± 2.4	75	39.4 ± 2.4	63	40.1 ± 2.0
	Control	102	37.0 ± 2.9	94	35.3 ± 2.7	74	40.0 ± 2.7	60	40.9 ± 2.5
Thrombocytes [1000/µL]	Intervention	103	239 ± 49	93	215 ± 44	75	243 ± 55	63	238 ± 56†
	Control	102	238 ± 46	94	227 ± 56	74	261 ± 58	60	263 ± 48†
Leukocytes [/nL]	Intervention	103	8.1 ± 2.0	93	8.9 ± 2.2#	75	5.5 ± 1.3	63	5.1 ± 1.1†
	Control	102	8.1 ± 1.6	94	9.6 ± 2.0#	74	5.9 ± 1.3	60	5.7 ± 1.3†
Quick/INR	Intervention	83	1.01 ± 0.06	89	1.00 ± 0.04	74	1.02 ± 0.05	64	1.03 ± 0.06
	Control	84	1.01 ± 0.07	92	0.99 ± 0.07	74	1.03 ± 0.06	60	1.03 ± 0.05
Quick [%]	Intervention	83	98 ± 8	89	101 ± 7	74	97 ± 8	64	96 ± 8
	Control	84	100 ± 9	92	103 ± 9	74	96 ± 8	60	96 ± 7
PTT [sec]	Intervention	83	33.1 ± 2.2	89	31.6 ± 2.2	74	35.3 ± 2.9	64	35.7 ± 3.1
	Control	84	32.8 ± 2.6	92	31.2 ± 2.0	74	34.9 ± 2.9	60	35.4 ± 2.9

\# Significantly different distribution between groups at 32nd week after Bonferroni-corrections (Mann-Whitney-U-Test) $p < 0.05$
† Significantly different distribution between groups 4 months pp after Bonferroni-corrections (Mann-Whitney-U-Test) $p < 0.05$
All intragroup-changes were significant over time (Friedman-Test)

Appendix

APPENDIX 2: Fatty acid composition of maternal RBCs during pregnancy and lactation

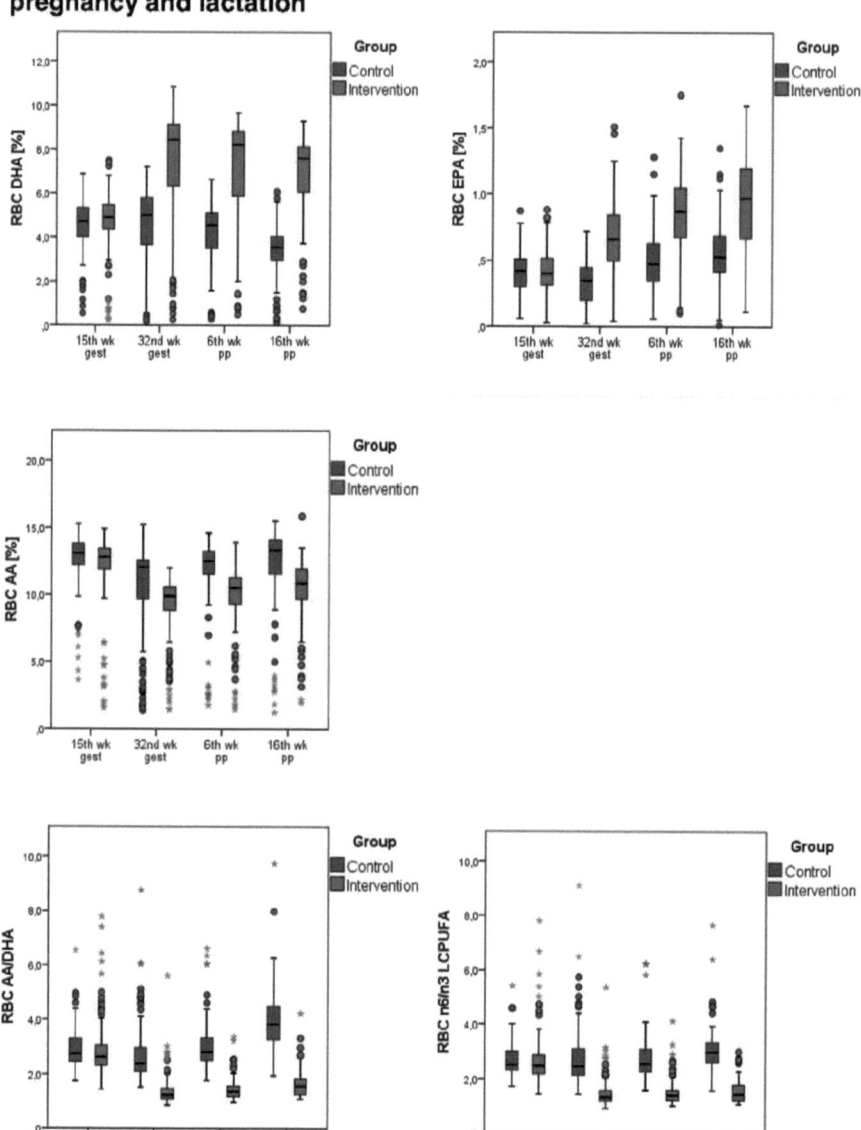

Data are presented as box-plots. Bottom and top edges of the box are located at 25th and 75th percentiles, center horizontal line is drawn at the median, whiskers mark the maximum and minimum. Outliners are shown as dots.

Appendix

APPENDIX 3: Fatty acid composition of maternal plasma PLs during pregnancy and lactation

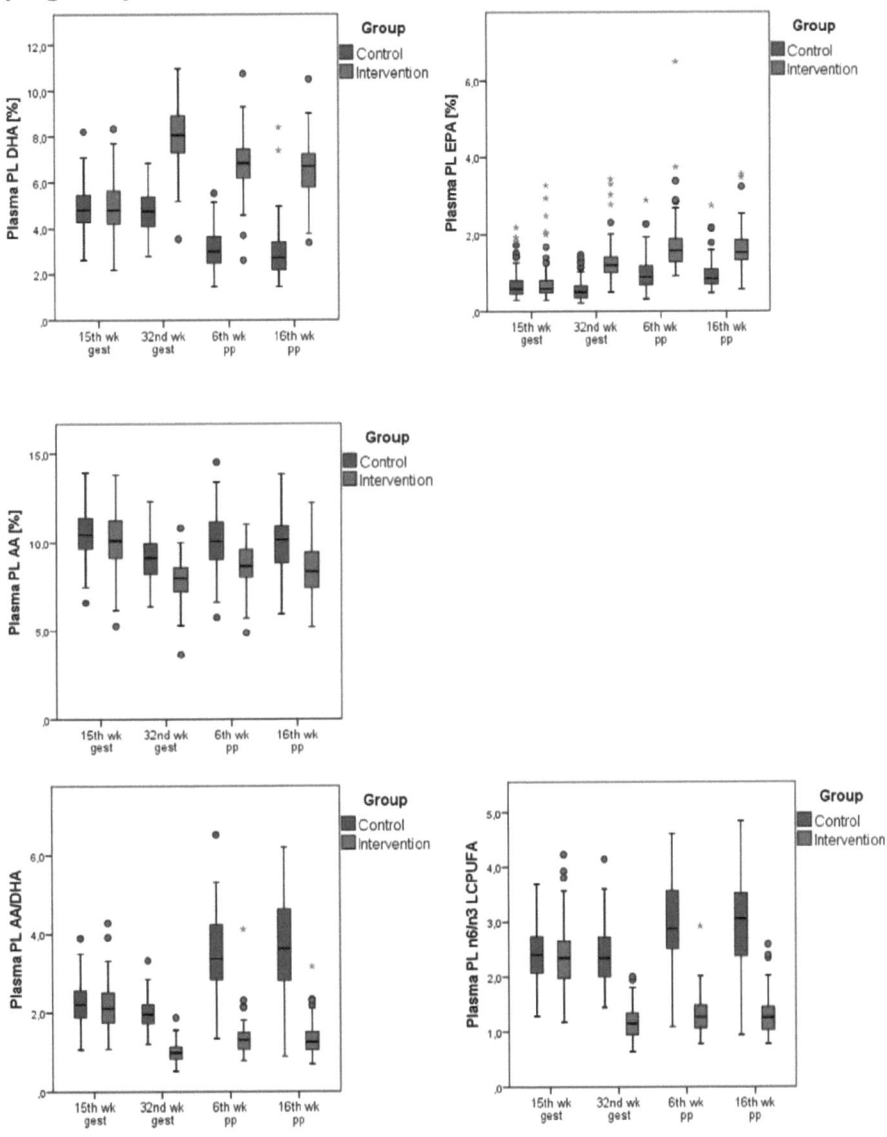

Data are presented as box-plots. Bottom and top edges of the box are located at 25th and 75th percentiles, center horizontal line is drawn at the median, whiskers mark the maximum and minimum. Outliners are shown as dots.

APPENDIX 4: Fatty acid composition of umbilical cord blood plasma PLs and RBCs at delivery

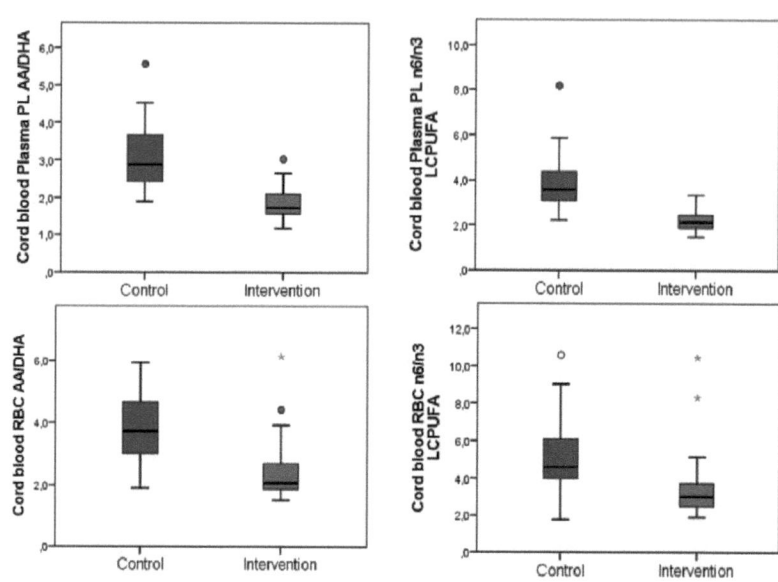

Data are presented as box-plots. Bottom and top edges of the box are located at 25th and 75th percentiles, center horizontal line is drawn at the median, whiskers mark the maximum and minimum. Outliners are shown as dots.

APPENDIX 5: Final adjusted multiple regression model and partial correlation coefficients on the effect of cord blood RBCs fatty acid status on infant growth and body fat mass at 1 year of age[1]

	n	cord RBCs DHA adj beta (95% CI)	r	cord RBCs AA/DHA adj beta (95% CI)	r	cord RBCs n-6/n-3 LCPUFAs adj beta (95% CI)	r
Weight [g]	122	10.25 (-62.33, 82.83)	0.16	-96.67 (-283.34, 90.00)	-0.18	-40.81 (-156.76, 75.15)	-0.16
Length [cm]	122	0.00 (-0.19, 0.19)	-0.12	-0.11 (-0.60, 0.38)	-0.14	0.00 (-0.31, 0.31)	-0.11
HC [cm]	122	0.08 (-0.04, 0.02)	0.23	-0.14 (-0.46, 0.18)	-0.20	-0.04 (-0.24, 0.15)	-0.17
BMI [kg/m^2]	122	0.02 (-0.08, 0.13)	0.10	-0.13 (-0.40, 0.14)	-0.10	-0.08 (-0.24, 0.09)	-0.11
PI [kg/m^3]	122	0.04 (-0.12, 0.19)	0.05	-0.16 (-0.56, 0.24)	-0.05	-0.11 (-0.36, 0.13)	-0.06
Sum 4 SFT [mm][2]	117	0.16 (-0.16, 0.48)	0.07	-0.49 (-1.33, 0.34)	-0.08	-0.17 (-0.69, 0.34)	-0.03
Fat mass [g][3]	117	13.33 (-18.77, 45.44)	0.12	-52.16 (-135.08, 30.77)	-0.14	-19.22 (-70.63, 32.19)	-0.10
Lean mass [g][3]	117	9.10 (-40.59, 58.78)	0.20	-72.95 (-201.14, 55.24)	-0.24	-38.52 (-117.76, 40.72)	-0.23
Fat mass [% bw][3]	117	0.12 (-0.10, 0.34)	0.07	-52.16 (-135.08, 30.77)	-0.14	-0.13 (-0.48, 0.23)	-0.04
SC sagittal [mm][2],[4]	112	0.00 (-0.01, 0.01)	0.01	-0.00 (-0.04, 0.02)	-0.03	0.00 (-0.02, 0.02)	-0.05
SC axial [mm][2],[5]	114	0.00 (-0.01, 0.01)	0.04	-0.01 (-0.04, 0.03)	-0.09	-0.00 (-0.02, 0.02)	-0.09
PP sagittal [mm][2],[4]	111	0.00 (0.0, 0.01)	0.03	-0.00 (-0.02, 0.01)	-0.03	-0.00 (-0.01, 0.01)	-0.04
Ratio SC/PP[6]	110	0.00 (-0.07, 0.07)	-0.05	-0.01 (-0.18, 0.16)	-0.10	0.02 (-0.08, 0.13)	0.13

[1] Data are presented as the regression coefficient of the fatty acid of interest (β) along with the (95% confidence interval) and the partial correlation coefficient according to Spearman (r) of the fatty acid of interest. At the time point of birth results were corrected for pregnancy duration, group, parity and sex. At 6 weeks pp, 4 month pp and 1 year pp, correction was performed for following variables: pregnancy duration, group, parity, sex, Ponderal index at birth and breastfeeding status at the respective time point. Breastfeeding status at 4 months was used in the analysis of the 1 year olds as it reflects the last time point of assessment. There were no consistently significant associations of any fatty acid with infant outcomes at 6 weeks pp and 4 months pp (data not shown). The stars indicate significant total model p-values of the (final) multivariable-adjusted analysis (F-test, ANCOVA, p< 0.05) and in the Spearman correlation coefficient (p< 0.05) in the analysis of the 1 year olds.

APPENDIX 6: Fatty acid composition of breast milk

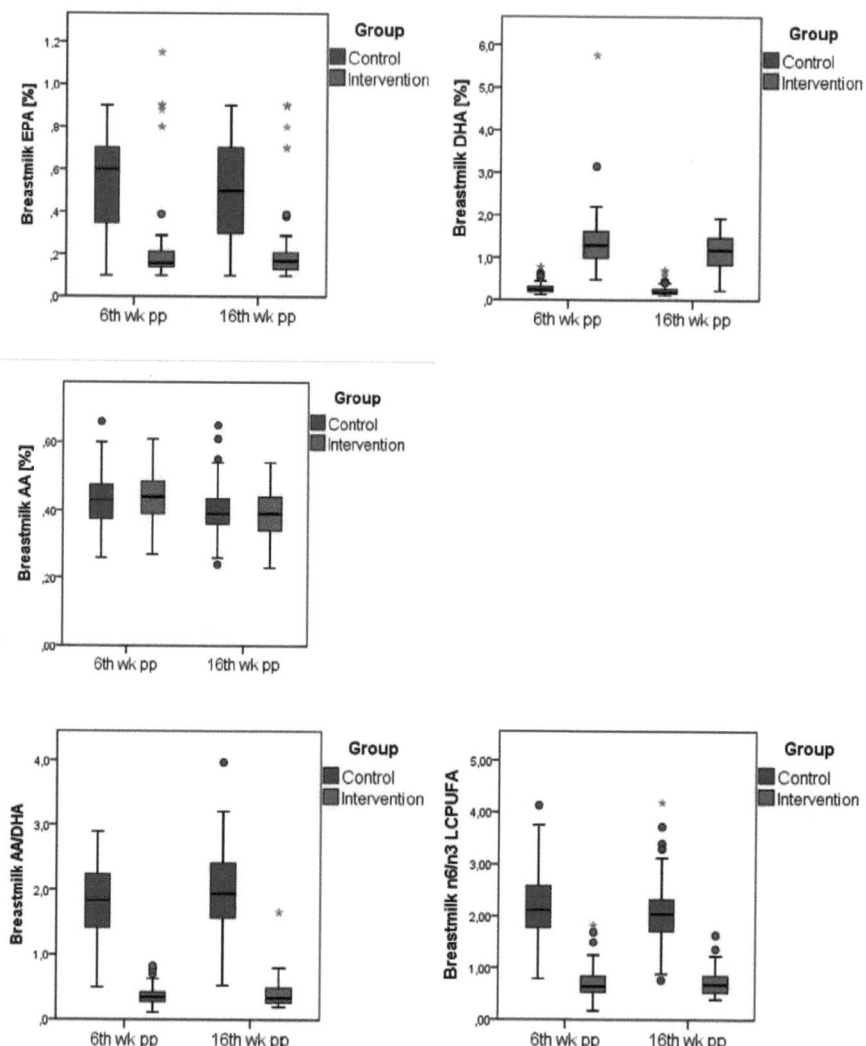

Data are presented as box-plots. Bottom and top edges of the box are located at 25th and 75th percentiles, center horizontal line is drawn at the median, whiskers mark the maximum and minimum. Outliners are shown as dots.

APPENDIX 7: Fatty acid composition of infant RBCs

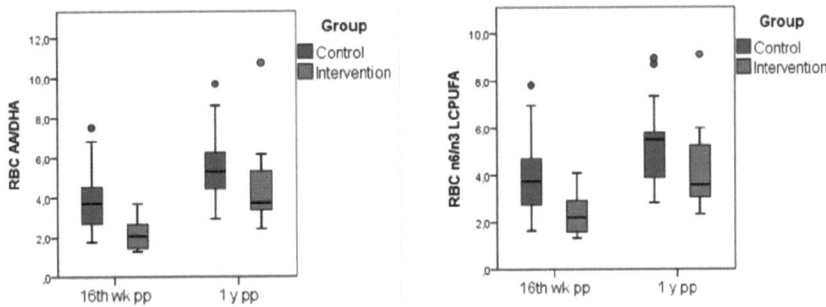

Data are presented as box-plots. Bottom and top edges of the box are located at 25th and 75th percentiles, center horizontal line is drawn at the median, whiskers mark the maximum and minimum. Outliners are shown as dots.

REFERENCES

1 **Adam O, Beringer C, Kless T, Lemmen C, Adam A, Wiseman M, Adam P, Klimmek R, Forth W** (2003). Anti-inflammatory effects of a low arachidonic acid diet and fish oil in patients with rheumatoid arthritis.
Rheumatol Int 23:27–36.

2 **Ailhaud G, Hauner H** (2004). Development of white adipose tissue. In "Handbook of Obesity, Etiology and Pathophysiology", 2nd edn. Marcel Dekker, New York-Basel.

3 **Ailhaud G, Guesnet P** (2004). Fatty acid composition of fats is an early determinant of childhood obesity: a short review and an opinion.
Obes Rev 5:21–26.

4 **Ailhaud G, Massiera F, Weill P, Legrand P, Alessandri J, Guesnet P** (2006). Temporal changes in dietary fats: role of n-6 polyunsaturated fatty acids in excessive adipose tissue development and relationship to obesity. Prog Lipid Res 45:203–236.

5 **Al MD, van Houwelingen AC, Kester AD, Hasaart TH, de J, Hornstra G** (1995). Maternal essential fatty acid patterns during normal pregnancy and their relationship to the neonatal essential fatty acid status.
Br J Nutr 74:55–68.

6 **Anandan C, Nurmatov U, Sheikh A** (2009). Omega 3 and 6 oils for primary prevention of allergic disease: systematic review and meta-analysis.
Allergy 64:840–848.

7 **Andersen AD, Michaelsen KF, Hellgren LI, Trolle E, Lauritzen L** (2011). A randomized controlled intervention with fish oil versus sunflower oil from 9 to 18 months of age: exploring changes in growth and skinfold thicknesses.
Pediatr Res 70(4):368-74. doi: 10.1038/pr.2011.593.

8   **Arai T, Kim H, Chiba H, Matsumoto A** (2009). Anti-obesity effect of fish oil and fish oil-fenofibrate combination in female KK mice. J Atheroscler Thromb 16:674–683.

9   **Armitage J, Taylor P, Poston L** (2005). Experimental models of developmental programming: consequences of exposure to an energy rich diet during development. J Physiol 565:3–8.

10 **Asserhoj M, Nehammer S, Matthiessen J, Michaelsen K, Lauritzen L** (2009). Maternal fish oil supplementation during lactation may adversely affect long-term blood pressure, energy intake, and physical activity of 7-year-old boys. J Nutr 139:298–304.

11 **Azain MJ** (2004). Role of fatty acids in adipocyte growth and development. J Anim Sci 82:916–924.

12 **Baird J, Fisher D, Lucas P, Kleijnen J, Roberts H, Law C** (2005). Being big or growing fast: systematic review of size and growth in infancy and later obesity. BMJ 331:929.

13 **Baum D, Beck RQ, Hammer LD, Brasel JA, Greenwood MR** (1986). Adipose tissue thymidine kinase activity in man. Pediatr Res 20:118–121.

14 **Beermann C, Mobius M, Winterling N, Schmitt J, Boehm G** (2005). sn-position determination of phospholipid-linked fatty acids derived from erythrocytes by liquid chromatography electrospray ionization ion-trap mass spectrometry. Lipids 40:211–218.

15 **Benfield LL, Fox KR, Peters DM, Blake H, Rogers I, Grant C, Ness A** (2008). Magnetic resonance imaging of abdominal adiposity in a large cohort of British children. Int J Obes (Lond) 32:91–99.

16 **Berghaus TM, Demmelmair H, Koletzko B** (2000). Essential fatty acids and their long-chain polyunsaturated metabolites in maternal and cord plasma triglycerides during late gestation. Biol Neonate 77:96–100.

17 **Bergmann L, Bergmann K, Haschke-Becher E, Richter R, Dudenhausen JW, Barclay D, Haschke F** (2007). Does maternal

docosahexaenoic acid supplementation during pregnancy and lactation lower BMI in late infancy? J Perinat Med 35:295–300.

18 **Bergmann L, Bergmann K, Richter R, Haschke-Becher E, Henrich W, Dudenhausen JW** (2012). Does docosahexaenoic acid (DHA) status in pregnancy have any impact on postnatal growth? Six-year follow-up of a prospective randomized double-blind monocenter study on low-dose DHA supplements. J Perinat Med, doi: 10.1515/jpm-2012-0080 (Epub ahead of print 15 January 2013).

19 **Blasbalg TL, Hibbeln JR, Ramsden CE, Majchrzak SF, Rawlings RR** (2011). Changes in consumption of omega-3 and omega-6 fatty acids in the United States during the 20th century. Am J Clin Nutr 93:950–962.

20 **Bligh EG, Dyer WJ** (1959). A rapid method of total lipid extraction and purification. Can J Biochem Physiol 37:911–917.

21 **Brambilla P, Bedogni G, Moreno LA, Goran MI, Gutin B, Fox KR, Peters DM, Barbeau P, De S, Pietrobelli A** (2006). Crossvalidation of anthropometry against magnetic resonance imaging for the assessment of visceral and subcutaneous adipose tissue in children. Int J Obes (Lond) 30:23–30.

22 **Brenna J, Varamini B, Jensen R, Diersen-Schade D, Boettcher J, Arterburn L** (2007). Docosahexaenoic and arachidonic acid concentrations in human breast milk worldwide. Am J Clin Nutr 85:1457–1464.

23 **Campbell K, Waters E, O'Meara S, Summerbell C** (2001). Interventions for preventing obesity in childhood. A systematic review.
Obesity Reviews 2:149–157.

24 **Campoy C, Escolano-Margarit M, Ramos R, Parrilla-Roure M, Csabi G, Beyer J, Ramirez-Tortosa M, Molloy A, Decsi T, Koletzko B** (2011). Effects of prenatal fish-oil and 5-methyltetrahydrofolate supplementation on cognitive development of children at 6.5 y of age. Am J Clin Nutr 94:1880S-1888S.

25 Campoy C, Escolano-Margarit MV, Anjos T, Szajewska H, Uauy R (2012). Omega 3 fatty acids on child growth, visual acuity and neurodevelopment.
Br J Nutr 107:S85.

26 Catalano PM, Drago NM, Amini SB (1995). Factors affecting fetal growth and body composition. Am J Obstet Gynecol 172:1459–1463.

27 Catalano PM, McIntyre HD, Cruickshank JK, McCance DR, Dyer AR, Metzger BE, Lowe LP, Trimble ER, Coustan DR, Hadden DR, Persson B, Hod M, Oats JJ (2012). The Hyperglycemia and Adverse Pregnancy Outcome Study: Associations of GDM and obesity with pregnancy outcomes. Diabetes Care 35:780–786.

28 Christie WW, Anne Urwin R (1995). Separation of lipid classes from plant tissues by high performance liquid chromatography on chemically bonded stationary phases. J. High Resol. Chromatogr 18:97–100.

29 Connor WE, Lowensohn R, Hatcher L (1996). Increased docosahexaenoic acid levels in human newborn infants by administration of sardines and fish oil during pregnancy. Lipids 31 Suppl:S183-7.

30 Coustan D, Lowe L, Metzger B, Dyer A (2010). The Hyperglycemia and Adverse Pregnancy Outcome (HAPO) study: paving the way for new diagnostic criteria for gestational diabetes mellitus.
Am J Obstet Gynecol 202:654.e1-6.

31 Crozier SR, Inskip HM, Godfrey KM, Cooper C, Harvey NC, Cole ZA, Robinson SM (2010). Weight gain in pregnancy and childhood body composition: findings from the Southampton Women's Survey.
Am J Clin Nutr 91:1745–1751.

32 Decsi T, Boehm G. Trans isomeric fatty acids are inversely related to the availability of long-chain polyunsaturated fatty acids in the perinatal period. Am J Clin Nutr (in press).

33 Del Prado M, Villalpando S, Elizondo A, Rodriguez M, Demmelmair H, Koletzko B (2001). Contribution of dietary and

newly formed arachidonic acid to human milk lipids in women eating a low-fat diet.
Am J Clin Nutr 74:242–247.

34 **Delgado-Noguera MF, Calvache JA, Bonfill Cosp X** (2010). Supplementation with long chain polyunsaturated fatty acids (LCPUFA) to breastfeeding mothers for improving child growth and development. Cochrane Database Syst Rev (12):CD007901.

35 **Deutsche Gesellschaft für Ernährung e.V.** Ratgeber: Wie ernähre ich mich in Schwangerschaft und Stillzeit? [German Nutrition Society. Booklet on healthy eating during pregnancy and breastfeeding.].

36 **Dirix C, Kester A, Hornstra G** (2009). Associations between neonatal birth dimensions and maternal essential and trans fatty acid contents during pregnancy and at delivery. Br J Nutr 101:399–407.

37 **Donahue S, Rifas-Shiman S, Gold D, Jouni Z, Gillman M, Oken E** (2011). Prenatal fatty acid status and child adiposity at age 3 y: results from a US pregnancy cohort. Am J Clin Nutr 93:780–788.

38 **Dunstan J, Mitoulas L, Dixon G, Doherty D, Hartmann P, Simmer K, Prescott S** (2007). The effects of fish oil supplementation in pregnancy on breast milk fatty acid composition over the course of lactation: a randomized controlled trial. Pediatr Res 62:689–694.

39 **Dunstan JA, Mori TA, Barden A, Beilin LJ, Holt PG, Calder PC, Taylor AL, Prescott SL** (2004). Effects of n-3 polyunsaturated fatty acid supplementation in pregnancy on maternal and fetal erythrocyte fatty acid composition.
Eur J Clin Nutr 58:429–437.

40 **Dunstan JA, Simmer K, Dixon G, Prescott SL** (2008). Cognitive assessment of children at age 2(1/2) years after maternal fish oil supplementation in pregnancy: a randomised controlled trial. Arch Dis Child Fetal Neonatal Ed 93:F45-50.

41 **Durmus B, Mook-Kanamori D, Holzhauer S, Hofman A, van der Beek EM, Boehm G, Steegers E, Jaddoe V** (2010). Growth in foetal life and infancy is associated with abdominal adiposity at the

age of 2 years: the generation R study. Clin Endocrinol (Oxf) 72:633–640.

42 Dziechciarz P, Horvath A, Szajewska H (2010). Effects of n-3 long-chain polyunsaturated fatty acid supplementation during pregnancy and/or lactation on neurodevelopment and visual function in children: a systematic review of randomized controlled trials. J Am Coll Nutr 29:443–454.

43 Ebbeling C, Pawlak D, Ludwig D (2002). Childhood obesity: public-health crisis, common sense cure. Lancet 360:473–482.

44 Elias SL, Innis SM (2001). Infant plasma trans, n-6, and n-3 fatty acids and conjugated linoleic acids are related to maternal plasma fatty acids, length of gestation, and birth weight and length. Am J Clin Nutr 73:807–814.

45 Ellis KJ (2007). Evaluation of body composition in neonates and infants. Semin Fetal Neonatal Med 12:87–91.

46 Escolano-Margarit M, Ramos R, Beyer J, Csabi G, Parrilla-Roure M, Cruz F, Perez-Garcia M, Hadders-Algra M, Gil A, Decsi T, Koletzko B, Campoy C (2011). Prenatal DHA status and neurological outcome in children at age 5.5 years are positively associated. J Nutr 141:1216–1223.

47 Fidler N, Sauerwald T, Pohl A, Demmelmair H, Koletzko B (2000). Docosahexaenoic acid transfer into human milk after dietary supplementation: a randomized clinical trial. J Lipid Res 41:1376–1383.

48 Fischer-Posovszky P, Wabitsch M (2004). Entwicklung und Funktion des Fettgewebes. Monatsschrift Kinderheilkunde 152:834-842.

49 Flachs P, Rossmeisl M, Bryhn M, Kopecky J (2009). Cellular and molecular effects of n-3 polyunsaturated fatty acids on adipose tissue biology and metabolism. Clin Sci (Lond) 116:1–16.

50 Fomon SJ, Haschke F, Ziegler EE, Nelson SE (1982). Body composition of reference children from birth to age 10 years. Am J Clin Nutr 35:1169–1175.

51 **Fox K, Peters D, Armstrong N, Sharpe P, Bell M** (1993). Abdominal fat deposition in 11-year-old children. Int J Obes Relat Metab Disord 17:11–16.

52 **Fraser A, Tilling K, Macdonald-Wallis C, Sattar N, Brion M, Benfield L, Ness A, Deanfield J, Hingorani A, Nelson SM, Smith GD, Lawlor DA** (2010). Association of maternal weight gain in pregnancy with offspring obesity and metabolic and vascular traits in childhood. Circulation 121:2557–2564.

53 **Gaillard D, Negrel R, Lagarde M, Ailhaud G** (1989). Requirement and role of arachidonic acid in the differentiation of pre-adipose cells.
Biochem J 257:389–397.

54 **Geer E, Shen W** (2009). Gender differences in insulin resistance, body composition, and energy balance. Gend Med 6 Suppl 1:60–75.

55 **German Society for Gynecology and Obstetrics eV.** Guidelines of the German Society for Gynecology and Obstetrics eV. Available via :http://www.dggg.de/leitlinien/aktuelle-leitlinien/ (cited 25 February 2011).

56 **Gillman M** (2010). Early infancy as a critical period for development of obesity and related conditions.
Nestle Nutr Workshop Ser Pediatr Program 65:13-20; discussion 20-4.

57 **Gillman M, Rifas-Shiman S, Kleinman K, Oken E, Rich-Edwards J, Taveras E** (2008). Developmental origins of childhood overweight: potential public health impact. Obesity (Silver Spring) 16:1651–1656.

58 **Gluckman PD, Hanson MA** (2008). Developmental and epigenetic pathways to obesity: an evolutionary-developmental perspective.
Int J Obes (Lond) 32 Suppl 7:S62-71.

59 **Haffner SM, Stern MP, Hazuda HP, Pugh J, Patterson JK** (1987). Do upper-body and centralized adiposity measure different aspects of regional body-fat distribution? Relationship to non-insulin-dependent diabetes mellitus, lipids, and lipoproteins. Diabetes 36:43–51.

60 **Hager A, Sjostrm L, Arvidsson B, Bjorntorp P, Smith U** (1977). Body fat and adipose tissue cellularity in infants: a longitudinal study. Metabolism 26:607–614.

61 **Haggarty P** (2002). Placental regulation of fatty acid delivery and its effect on fetal growth--a review. Placenta 23 Suppl A:S28-38.

62 **Hauner H, Brunner S, Amann-Gassner U**. The role of dietary fatty acids for early human adipose tissue growth. Am J Clin Nutr (in press).

63 **Hauner H, Wabitsch M** (1989). Proliferation and differentiation of adipose tissue derived stroma-vascular cells from children at different ages. In: Björntrop P, Rössner S, eds. Obesity in Europe 88: Proceedings of the 1st European Congress on Obesity. London-Paris, Libbey:195-200.

64 **Hauner H, Much D, Vollhardt C, Brunner S, Schmid D, Sedlmeier E, Heimberg E, Schuster T, Zimmermann A, Schneider KM, Bader BL, Amann-Gassner U** (2012). Effect of reducing the n-6:n-3 long-chain PUFA ratio during pregnancy and lactation on infant adipose tissue growth within the first year of life: an open-label randomized controlled trial. Am J Clin Nutr 95:383–394.

65 **Hauner H, Vollhardt C, Schneider KT, Zimmermann A, Schuster T, Amann-Gassner U** (2009). The impact of nutritional fatty acids during pregnancy and lactation on early human adipose tissue development. Rationale and design of the INFAT study. Ann Nutr Metab 54:97–103.

66 **Helland I, Smith L, Blomen B, Saarem K, Saugstad O, Drevon C** (2008). Effect of supplementing pregnant and lactating mothers with n-3 very-long-chain fatty acids on children's IQ and body mass index at 7 years of age. Pediatrics 122:e472-9.

67 **Helland I, Smith L, Saarem K, Saugstad O, Drevon C** (2003). Maternal supplementation with very-long-chain n-3 fatty acids during pregnancy and lactation augments children's IQ at 4 years of age. Pediatrics 111:e39-44.

68 **Helland IB, Saugstad OD, Smith L, Saarem K, Solvoll K, Ganes T, Drevon CA** (2001). Similar Effects on Infants of n-3 and n-6 Fatty Acids Supplementation to Pregnant and Lactating Women. Pediatrics 108:e82.

69 **Heslehurst N, Rankin J, Wilkinson JR, Summerbell CD** (2010). A nationally representative study of maternal obesity in England, UK: trends in incidence and demographic inequalities in 619 323 births, 1989-2007.
Int J Obes (Lond) 34:420–428.

70 **Holzhauer S, Zwijsen R, Jaddoe V, Boehm G, Moll H, Mulder P, Kleyburg-Linkers V, Hofman A, Witteman J** (2009). Sonographic assessment of abdominal fat distribution in infancy. Eur J Epidemiol 24:521–529.

71 **Hull H, Thornton J, Ji Y, Paley C, Rosenn B, Mathews P, Navder K, Yu A, Dorsey K, Gallagher D** (2011). Higher infant body fat with excessive gestational weight gain in overweight women.
Am J Obstet Gynecol 205:211.e1-7.

72 **Innis S, Friesen R** (2008). Essential n-3 fatty acids in pregnant women and early visual acuity maturation in term infants. Am J Clin Nutr 87:548–557.

73 **Jans LA, Giltay EJ, van der Does AJ** (2010). The efficacy of n-3 fatty acids DHA and EPA (fish oil) for perinatal depression. Br J Nutr 104:1577–1585.

74 **Jensen C, Voigt R, Prager T, Zou Y, Fraley J, Rozelle J, Turcich M, Llorente A, Anderson R, Heird W** (2005). Effects of maternal docosahexaenoic acid intake on visual function and neurodevelopment in breastfed term infants. Am J Clin Nutr 82:125–132.

75 **Knittle JL, Timmers K, Ginsberg-Fellner F, Brown RE, Katz DP** (1979). The growth of adipose tissue in children and adolescents. Cross-sectional and longitudinal studies of adipose cell number and size. J Clin Invest 63:239–246.

76 **Koo W, Walters J, Hockman E** (2004). Body composition in neonates: relationship between measured and derived

anthropometry with dual-energy X-ray absorptiometry measurements. Pediatr Res 56:694–700.

77 **Krauss-Etschmann S, Shadid R, Campoy C, Hoster E, Demmelmair H, Jimenez M, Gil A, Rivero M, Veszpremi B, Decsi T, Koletzko B** (2007). Effects of fish-oil and folate supplementation of pregnant women on maternal and fetal plasma concentrations of docosahexaenoic acid and eicosapentaenoic acid: a European randomized multicenter trial.
Am J Clin Nutr 85:1392–1400.

78 **Kris-Etherton PM, Taylor DS, Yu-Poth S, Huth P, Moriarty K, Fishell V, Hargrove RL, Zhao G, Etherton TD** (2000). Polyunsaturated fatty acids in the food chain in the United States.
Am J Clin Nutr 71:179S-88S.

79 **Kromeyer-Hauschild K, Wabitsch M, Kunze D, Geller F, Geiß, H. C., Hesse V, Hippel A von, Jaeger U, Johnsen D, Korte W, Menner K, Müller G, Müller JM, Niemann-Pilatus A, Remer T, Schaefer F, Wittchen H, Zabransky S, Zellner K, Ziegler A, Hebebrand J** (2001). Perzentile für den Body-mass-Index für das Kindes- und Jugendalter unter Heranziehung verschiedener deutscher Stichproben.
Monatsschrift Kinderheilkunde 149:807–818.

80 **Kuipers RS, Luxwolda MF, Offringa PJ, Boersma ER, Dijck-Brouwer DA, Muskiet FA** (2012). Fetal intrauterine whole body linoleic, arachidonic and docosahexaenoic acid contents and accretion rates. Prostaglandins Leukot Essent Fatty Acids 86(1-2):13–20.

81 **Kuk J, Lee S, Heymsfield S, Ross R** (2005). Waist circumference and abdominal adipose tissue distribution: influence of age and sex.
Am J Clin Nutr 81:1330–1334.

82 **Kurth B, Schaffrath R** (2010). Übergewicht und Adipositas bei Kindern und Jugendlichen in Deutschland. Bundesgesundheitsblatt Gesundheitsforschung Gesundheitsschutz 53:643–652.

83 **Lapillonne A, Clarke S, Heird W** (2003). Plausible mechanisms for effects of long-chain polyunsaturated fatty acids on growth. J Pediatr 143:S9-16.

84 Larqué E, Gil-Sánchez A, Prieto-Sánchez MT, Koletzko B (2012). Omega 3 fatty acids, gestation and pregnancy outcomes. Br J Nutr 107:S77.

85 **Lauritzen L, Hoppe C, Straarup E, Michaelsen K** (2005a). Maternal fish oil supplementation in lactation and growth during the first 2.5 years of life. Pediatr Res 58:235–242.

86 **Lauritzen L, Jorgensen M, Mikkelsen T, Skovgaard I, Straarup E, Olsen S, Hoy C, Michaelsen K** (2004). Maternal fish oil supplementation in lactation: effect on visual acuity and n-3 fatty acid content of infant erythrocytes.
Lipids 39:195–206.

87 **Lauritzen L, Jorgensen M, Olsen S, Straarup E, Michaelsen K** (2005b). Maternal fish oil supplementation in lactation: effect on developmental outcome in breast-fed infants. Reprod Nutr Dev 45:535–547.

88 **Lepage G, Roy CC** (1984). Improved recovery of fatty acid through direct transesterification without prior extraction or purification.
J Lipid Res 25:1391–1396.

89 **Liu KH, Chan YL, Chan WB, Kong WL, Kong MO, Chan JC** (2003). Sonographic measurement of mesenteric fat thickness is a good correlate with cardiovascular risk factors: comparison with subcutaneous and preperitoneal fat thickness, magnetic resonance imaging and anthropometric indexes.
Int J Obes Relat Metab Disord 27:1267–1273.

90 **Madsen L, Petersen R, Kristiansen K** (2005). Regulation of adipocyte differentiation and function by polyunsaturated fatty acids.
Biochim Biophys Acta 1740:266–286.

91 **Makrides M, Duley L, Olsen SF** (2006). Marine oil, and other prostaglandin precursor, supplementation for pregnancy uncomplicated by pre-eclampsia or intrauterine growth restriction. Cochrane Database Syst Rev 3:CD003402.

92 **Makrides M, Gibson R, McPhee A, Yelland L, Quinlivan J, Ryan P** (2010). Effect of DHA supplementation during pregnancy on maternal depression and neurodevelopment of young children: a randomized controlled trial.

JAMA 304:1675–1683.

93   **Makrides M, Neumann MA, Gibson RA** (1996). Effect of maternal docosahexaenoic acid (DHA) supplementation on breast milk composition.
Eur J Clin Nutr 50:352–357.

94   **Malcolm CA** (2003). Maternal docosahexaenoic acid supplementation during pregnancy and visual evoked potential development in term infants: a double blind, prospective, randomised trial.
Archives of Disease in Childhood - Fetal and Neonatal Edition 88:383F.

95   **Mamun A, Kinarivala M, O'Callaghan M, Williams G, Najman J, Callaway L** (2010). Associations of excess weight gain during pregnancy with long-term maternal overweight and obesity: evidence from 21 y postpartum follow-up. Am J Clin Nutr 91:1336–1341.

96   **Massiera F, Saint-Marc P, Seydoux J, Murata T, Kobayashi T, Narumiya S, Guesnet P, Amri E, Negrel R, Ailhaud G** (2003). Arachidonic acid and prostacyclin signaling promote adipose tissue development: a human health concern? J Lipid Res 44:271–279.

97   **Max-Rubner-Institut** (2008). Nationale Verzehrsstudie II. Max Rubner-Institut, Bundesforschungsinstitut für Ernährung und Lebensmittel, Karlsruhe.

98   **McLaren DS** (1987). A fresh look at some perinatal growth and nutritional standards. World Rev Nutr Diet 49:87–120.

99   **Molto-Puigmarti C, Plat J, Mensink R, Muller A, Jansen E, Zeegers M, Thijs C** (2010). FADS1 FADS2 gene variants modify the association between fish intake and the docosahexaenoic acid proportions in human milk.
Am J Clin Nutr 91:1368–1376.

100 **Moss A, Klenk J, Simon K, Thaiss H, Reinehr T, Wabitsch M** (2012). Declining prevalence rates for overweight and obesity in German children starting school. Eur J Pediatr 171:289–299.

101 **Mook-Kanamori DO, Holzhauer S, Hollestein LM, Durmus B, Manniesing R, Koek M, Boehm G, van der Beek EM, Hofman A,**

Witteman JC, Lequin MH, Jaddoe VW (2009). Abdominal fat in children measured by ultrasound and computed tomography. Ultrasound Med Biol. 35(12):1938-46.

102 **Muhlhausler B, Gibson R, Makrides M** (2010). Effect of long-chain polyunsaturated fatty acid supplementation during pregnancy or lactation on infant and child body composition: a systematic review.
Am J Clin Nutr 92:857–863.

103 **Muhlhausler B, Miljkovic D, Fong L, Xian C, Duthoit E, Gibson R** (2011a). Maternal omega-3 supplementation increases fat mass in male and female rat offspring. Front Genet 2:48.

104 **Muhlhausler BS, Gibson RA, Makrides M** (2011b). The effect of maternal omega-3 long-chain polyunsaturated fatty acid (n-3 LCPUFA) supplementation during pregnancy and/or lactation on body fat mass in the offspring: a systematic review of animal studies.
Prostaglandins Leukot Essent Fatty Acids 85:83–88.

105 **Nehring I, Schmoll S, Beyerlein A, Hauner H, von Kries** (2011). Gestational weight gain and long-term postpartum weight retention: a meta-analysis.
Am J Clin Nutr 94:1225–1231.

106 **Nelson S, Matthews P, Poston L** (2010). Maternal metabolism and obesity: modifiable determinants of pregnancy outcome.
Hum Reprod Update 16:255–275.

107 **Ogden C, Carroll M, Kit B, Flegal K** (2012). Prevalence of obesity and trends in body mass index among US children and adolescents, 1999-2010.
JAMA 307:483–490.

108 **Oka R, Miura K, Sakurai M, Nakamura K, Yagi K, Miyamoto S, Moriuchi T, Mabuchi H, Yamagishi M, Takeda Y, Hifumi S, Inazu A, Nohara A, Kawashiri M, Kobayashi J** (2009). Comparison of waist circumference with body mass index for predicting abdominal adipose tissue.
Diabetes Res Clin Pract 83:100–105.

109 **Oken E, Gillman M** (2003). Fetal origins of obesity. Obes Res 11:496–506.

110 **Olds TS** (2009). One million skinfolds: secular trends in the fatness of young people 1951-2004. Eur J Clin Nutr 63:934–946.

111 **Olhager E, Flinke E, Hannerstad U, Forsum E** (2003). Studies on human body composition during the first 4 months of life using magnetic resonance imaging and isotope dilution. Pediatr Res 54:906–912.

112 **Olsen SF, Hansen HS, Sorensen TI, Jensen B, Secher NJ, Sommer S, Knudsen LB** (1986). Intake of marine fat, rich in (n-3)-polyunsaturated fatty acids, may increase birthweight by prolonging gestation. Lancet 2:367–369.

113 **Olsen SF, Sorensen JD, Secher NJ, Hedegaard M, Henriksen TB, Hansen HS, Grant A** (1992). Randomised controlled trial of effect of fish-oil supplementation on pregnancy duration. Lancet 339:1003–1007.

114 **Onis M de, Blossner M, Borghi E** (2010). Global prevalence and trends of overweight and obesity among preschool children. Am J Clin Nutr 92:1257–1264.

115 **Oosting A, Kegler D, Boehm G, Jansen H, van de Heijning BJ, van der Beek EM** (2010). N-3 long-chain polyunsaturated fatty acids prevent excessive fat deposition in adulthood in a mouse model of postnatal nutritional programming. Pediatr Res 68:494–499.

116 **Owens S, Litaker M, Allison J, Riggs S, Ferguson M, Gutin B** (1999). Prediction of visceral adipose tissue from simple anthropometric measurements in youths with obesity. Obes Res 7:16–22.

117 **Pedersen L, Lauritzen L, Brasholt M, Buhl T, Bisgaard H** (2012). Polyunsaturated fatty acid content of mother´s milk is associated with childhood body composition. Pediatr Res, doi: 10.1038/pr.2012.127 (Epub ahead of print 12 December 2012).

118 **Peneau S, Rouchaud A, Rolland-Cachera M, Arnault N, Hercberg S, Castetbon K** (2011). Body size and growth from birth to 2 years and risk of overweight at 7-9 years. Int J Pediatr Obes 6:e162-9.

119 **Pietilainen KH, Kaprio J, Rasanen M, Winter T, Rissanen A, Rose RJ** (2001). Tracking of body size from birth to late adolescence: contributions of birth length, birth weight, duration of gestation, parents' body size, and twinship. Am J Epidemiol 154:21–29.

120 **Poissonnet CM, Burdi AR, Bookstein FL** (1983). Growth and development of human adipose tissue during early gestation. Early Hum Dev 8:1–11.

121 **Poissonnet CM, Burdi AR, Garn SM** (1984). The chronology of adipose tissue appearance and distribution in the human fetus. Early Hum Dev 10:1–11.

122 **Rump P, Mensink RP, Kester AD, Hornstra G** (2001). Essential fatty acid composition of plasma phospholipids and birth weight: a study in term neonates. Am J Clin Nutr 73:797–806.

123 **Rytter D, Christensen JH, Bech BH, Schmidt EB, Henriksen TB, Olsen SF** (2012). The effect of maternal fish oil supplementation during the last trimester of pregnancy on blood pressure, heart rate and heart rate variability in the 19-year-old offspring. Br J Nutr:1–9.

124 **Brunner S, Much D, Amann-Gassner U, Hauner H (2011).** Fischöl in der Schwangerschaft? – Neue Erkenntnisse. Adipositas – Ursachen, Folgeerkrankungen, Therapie (Vol. 5): Heft 4.

125 **Salans LB, Cushman SW, Weismann RE** (1973). Studies of human adipose tissue. Adipose cell size and number in nonobese and obese patients.
J Clin Invest 52:929–941.

126 **Sanders TA** (2000). Polyunsaturated fatty acids in the food chain in Europe. Am J Clin Nutr 71:176S-8S.

127 **Schack-Nielsen L, Michaelsen KF, Gamborg M, Mortensen EL, Sorensen TI** (2010). Gestational weight gain in relation to offspring body mass index and obesity from infancy through adulthood. Int J Obes (Lond) 34:67–74.

128 **Schmelzle H, Fusch C** (2002). Body fat in neonates and young infants: validation of skinfold thickness versus dual-energy X-ray absorptiometry. Am J Clin Nutr 76:1096–1100.

129 **Singh AS, Mulder C, Twisk JW, van Mechelen W, Chinapaw MJ** (2008). Tracking of childhood overweight into adulthood: a systematic review of the literature. Obes Rev 9:474–488.

130 **Sjostrom L, William-Olsson T** (1981). Prospective studies on adipose tissue development in man. Int J Obes 5:597–604.

131 **Skouteris H, Hartley-Clark L, McCabe M, Milgrom J, Kent B, Herring SJ, Gale J** (2010). Preventing excessive gestational weight gain: a systematic review of interventions. Obes Rev 11:757–768.

132 **Smit EN, Martini IA, Mulder H, Boersma ER, Muskiet FA** (2002). Estimated biological variation of the mature human milk fatty acid composition. Prostaglandins Leukot Essent Fatty Acids 66:549–555.

133 **Soyama A, Nishikawa T, Ishizuka T, Ito H, Saito J, Yagi K, Saito Y** (2005). Clinical usefulness of the thickness of preperitoneal and subcutaneous fat layer in the abdomen estimated by ultrasonography for diagnosing abdominal obesity in each type of impaired glucose tolerance in man. Endocr J 52:229–236.

134 **Spalding KL, Arner E, Westermark PO, Bernard S, Buchholz BA, Bergmann O, Blomqvist L, Hoffstedt J, Näslund E, Britton T, Concha H, Hassan M, Rydén M, Frisén J, Arner P** (2008). Dynamics of fat cell turnover in humans. Nature 453:783–787.

135 **Stratz W** (1902). Der Körper des Kindes. Emke Verlag, Stuttgart.

136 **Suzuki R, Watanabe S, Hirai Y, Akiyama K, Nishide T, Matsushima Y, Murayama H, Ohshima H, Shinomiya M, Shirai K** (1993). Abdominal wall fat index, estimated by ultrasonography, for assessment of the ratio of visceral fat to subcutaneous fat in the abdomen. Am J Med 95:309–314.

137 **Szajewska H, Horvath A, Koletzko B** (2006). Effect of n-3 long-chain polyunsaturated fatty acid supplementation of women with

low-risk pregnancies on pregnancy outcomes and growth measures at birth: a meta-analysis of randomized controlled trials. Am J Clin Nutr 83:1337–1344.

138 **Tamura A, Mori T, Hara Y, Komiyama A** (2000). Preperitoneal fat thickness in childhood obesity: association with serum insulin concentration.
Pediatr Int 42:155–159.

139 **Tanaka Y, Kikuchi T, Nagasaki K, Hiura M, Ogawa Y, Uchiyama M** (2005). Lower birth weight and visceral fat accumulation are related to hyperinsulinemia and insulin resistance in obese Japanese children. Hypertens Res 28:529–536.

140 **Tanentsapf I, Heitmann B, Adegboye A** (2011). Systematic review of clinical trials on dietary interventions to prevent excessive weight gain during pregnancy among normal weight, overweight and obese women.
BMC Pregnancy Childbirth 11:81.

141 **Taveras E, Rifas-Shiman S, Belfort M, Kleinman K, Oken E, Gillman M** (2009). Weight status in the first 6 months of life and obesity at 3 years of age. Pediatrics 123:1177–1183.

142 **Taylor PD, Poston L** (2007). Developmental programming of obesity in mammals. Exp Physiol 92:287–298.

143 **van Eijsden M, Hornstra G, van der Wal MF, Vrijkotte TG, Bonsel GJ** (2008). Maternal n-3, n-6, and trans fatty acid profile early in pregnancy and term birth weight: a prospective cohort study. Am J Clin Nutr 87:887–895.

144 **van Houwelingen AC, Ham EC, Hornstra G** (1999). The female docosahexaenoic acid status related to the number of completed pregnancies. Lipids 34:S229.

145 **van Houwelingen AC, Søsrensen JD, Hornstra G, Simonis MM, Boris J, Olsen SF, Secher NJ** (1995). Essential fatty acid status in neonates after fish-oil supplementation during late pregnancy. BJN 74:723.

146 **Velzing-Aarts FV, van der Klis FR, van der Dijs FP, van Beusekom CM, Landman H, Capello JJ, Muskiet FA** (2001). Effect of three low-dose fish oil supplements, administered during

pregnancy, on neonatal long-chain polyunsaturated fatty acid status at birth. Prostaglandins Leukot Essent Fatty Acids 65:51–57.

147 **Voigt M, Straube S, Zygmunt M, Krafczyk B, Schneider KT, Briese V** (2008). Obesity and pregnancy--a risk profile. Z Geburtshilfe Neonatol 212:201–205.

148 **Wang Y, Beydoun M, Liang L, Caballero B, Kumanyika S** (2008). Will all Americans become overweight or obese? estimating the progression and cost of the US obesity epidemic. Obesity (Silver Spring) 16:2323–2330.

149 **Wells JC, Fewtrell MS** (2006). Measuring body composition. Arch Dis Child 91:612–617.

150 **Weseler A, Dirix C, Bruins M, Hornstra G** (2008). Dietary arachidonic acid dose-dependently increases the arachidonic acid concentration in human milk. J Nutr 138:2190–2197.

151 **Weststrate JA, Deurenberg P** (1989). Body composition in children: proposal for a method for calculating body fat percentage from total body density or skinfold-thickness measurements. Am J Clin Nutr 50:1104–1115.

152 **Weststrate JA, Deurenberg P, van Tinteren H** (1989). Indices of body fat distribution and adiposity in Dutch children from birth to 18 years of age. Int J Obes 13:465–477.

153 **Widdowsen EM** (1950). Chemical composition of newly born mammals. Nature 166:626–628.

154 **WHO | WHO Forum and Technical Meeting on Population-based Prevention Strategies for Childhood Obesity. Geneva, Switzerland 15-17 December 2009.** Available via http://www.who.int/dietphysicalactivity/childhood/report/en/index.html. Accessed 20 Feb 2012.

155 **Wright CM, Emmett PM, Ness AR, Reilly JJ, Sherriff A** (2010). Tracking of obesity and body fatness through mid-childhood. Arch Dis Child 95:612–617.

156 **Yuhas R, Pramuk K, Lien EL** (2006). Human milk fatty acid composition from nine countries varies most in DHA. Lipids 41:851–858.

157 **Zhou SJ, Yelland L, McPhee AJ, Quinlivan J, Gibson RA, Makrides M** (2012). Fish-oil supplementation in pregnancy does not reduce the risk of gestational diabetes or preeclampsia. Am J Clin Nutr.

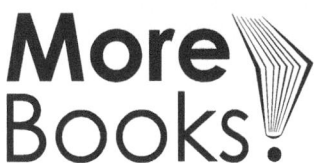

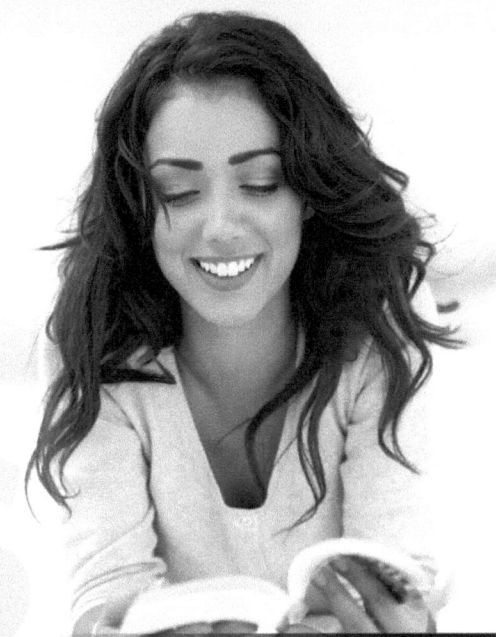

i want morebooks!

Buy your books fast and straightforward online - at one of world's fastest growing online book stores! Environmentally sound due to Print-on-Demand technologies.

Buy your books online at
www.get-morebooks.com

Kaufen Sie Ihre Bücher schnell und unkompliziert online – auf einer der am schnellsten wachsenden Buchhandelsplattformen weltweit! Dank Print-On-Demand umwelt- und ressourcenschonend produziert.

Bücher schneller online kaufen
www.morebooks.de

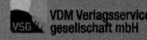 VDM Verlagsservicegesellschaft mbH
Heinrich-Böcking-Str. 6-8   Telefon: +49 681 3720 174   info@vdm-vsg.de
D - 66121 Saarbrücken   Telefax: +49 681 3720 1749 www.vdm-vsg.de

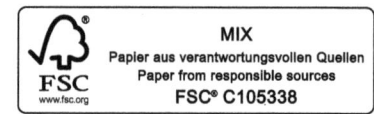

Printed by Books on Demand GmbH, Norderstedt / Germany